Worthy IN HIS Eyes

Looking Beyond

the

Reflection in the Mirror

KATHLEEN M. PRITCHARD

WORTHY IN HIS EYES
Copyright © 2012 by Kathleen M. Pritchard

Unless otherwise noted, scriptures are taken from THE HOLY BIBLE, NEW INTERNATIONAL VERSION®, NIV® Copyright © 1973, 1978, 1984, 2011 by Biblica, Inc.™ Used by permission. All rights reserved worldwide. • Scriptures marked "CEV" are taken from Contemporary English Version® Copyright © 1995 American Bible Society. All rights reserved. • Scripture marked "The Message" taken from The Message. Copyright © 1993, 1994, 1995, 1996, 2000, 2001, 2002. Used by permission of NavPress Publishing Group.

ISBN:978-1-77069-441-5

Printed in Canada.

Word Alive Press
131 Cordite Road, Winnipeg, MB R3W 1S1
www.wordalivepress.ca

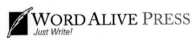

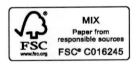

MIX
Paper from
responsible sources
FSC® C016245

Library and Archives Canada Cataloguing in Publication
Pritchard, Kathleen M., 1960-
    Worthy in his eyes : looking beyond the reflection
in the mirror / Kathleen Pritchard.
ISBN 978-1-77069-441-5
    1. Pritchard, Kathleen M., 1960-. 2. Brain--Wounds and injuries--Patients--Biography. 3. Brain--Wounds and injuries--Patients--Religious life. 4. Brain--Wounds and injuries--Patients--Rehabilitation. I. Title.
RJ496.B7P75 2012   617.4'81044092   C2011-908432-5

Table of Contents

WITH DEEP APPRECIATION TO...

MY LORD AND SAVIOUR, JESUS CHRIST, FOR WASHING MY EYES WITH THE salve of truth, enabling me to celebrate abundant living, because I am *Worthy in Your Eyes.*

My son Kris—Your contagious sense of humour opens up skies of sunshine on cloudy and rainy days. I am still "Mom" to you, and your unconditional love and acceptance makes me almost forget I have a disability. I love you for that priceless gift.

My daughter Krystal—You have grown me in many ways, and through you I have learned a great deal about myself. You have intensified my awareness of how deep a mother's love can anchor itself within her heart.

My precious mother, Margaret—Words cannot even begin to express the gratitude in my heart to you for the greatest gift a parent can give a child, the truth of the gospel which leads to eternal life. You have profoundly influenced my life, and I am so grateful for all the blessings you have brought into my world since I was born.

My Auntie Kathie—Thank you for your encouragement, support, and excitement about this book. Your enthusiasm to promote my book to "every store in the city" fills my heart with gratitude.

Our families—I love you for your thoughtfulness and kindness when we get together. I appreciate the efforts made to accommodate some of my limitations.

My precious friend and mentor Shirley—Endless times you have nudged me, gently reminding me to be obedient to God by pressing on with this book. Your prayers, encouragement, and wisdom (both spiritual and practical) have helped me through some really tough times. Thanks for our special Internet tea and prayer times. Also, to your husband (and my very favourite pastor) Dave, it was you whom God used to fully reawaken the one thing in my life I missed so terribly—that uninhibited twinkle in my eye. Thank you so much for being you!

My cherished friend Jan—Your friendship, love, encouragement, support and prayers have remained solid for two decades. You are a true prayer warrior. How grateful I am that we are "forever" friends. You've always been there for me; now it's my turn to be there for you.

My faithful friend Kitty—I am grateful for your friendship, encouragement, enormous support and very tangible help. Without you, I would *never* be able to accomplish what I do now. Our "game" always triggers a wonderful sense of imagination *and* a great giggle! You are a gem.

Our treasured friends, Don and Lee—As couples, we have shared special times together for twenty years. Your support, love, humour and prayer have helped us continue to move forward after our lives took a drastic turn. We love you for being there.

My vibrant, spontaneous friend Susan—How grateful I am God knew we would be a perfect fit as friends not so long ago. I love your laugh, your strength, and your love for words! You are a jewel in my treasure chest.

Debbie Dee—Your focus to provide education and awareness of acquired brain injuries is admirable, and those of us who live with the disability highly respect the work you do. I am personally grateful for your strength, wisdom, encouragement and contagious smile. Thank you so much for your willingness to give me feedback regarding my book.

Linda Wegner—Your trained eye and unwavering belief in my writing, and my story, gave me the courage to begin my publishing journey. Thank you for introducing me to Word Alive Press.

My editor, Tom Buller—You are a Barnabas (encourager). You worked with my disability, and made the editing process enjoyable! Thank you for your professionalism and light-hearted sense of humour.

Word Alive Press—Caroline Schmidt, thank you for your enthusiasm and guidance as I began my publishing journey. I appreciate every person involved in the process of publishing this book.

To *so* many others who have encouraged Kip and me—Thank you for your tremendous support, enquiring about my progress with this book, urging me to see it through all the way because "more people need to learn about this invisible disability."

Dedication

This book is dedicated to my cherished husband, Kip. Your willingness to adapt to major life changes cemented the solid foundation we had prior to my car accident, empowering us to discover fullness of life once again.

Your unconditional love has dried many a tear, encouraged me, induced humour and made me fully treasure the sacred vows we made to God, and each other, thirty-two years ago. Your strong faith and trust in the Lord enabled Him to shine through even the darkest nights.

Through so much, we have not only remained in love, we have grown deeper in love. Because of you, I am free to be me. For these gifts, I thank you with all of my heart.

PREFACE

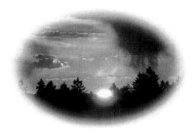

Worth How Much?

"For you created my inmost being; you knit me together in my mother's womb. I praise you because I am fearfully and wonderfully made; your works are wonderful, I know that full well. My frame was not hidden from you when I was made in the secret place. When I was woven together in the depths of the earth, your eyes saw my unformed body. All the days ordained for me were written in your book before one of them came to be."
(Psalm 139:13–16)

FRANTICALLY, I HAD CALLED MY HUSBAND WHO WAS MEETING WITH A client in their home. "You've got to come back right away; I can't understand what is going on! There are two clients in the shop and I can't make sense of what they are saying! Please, please come back right away!"

A few days earlier, a car had slammed into the rear of my van, throwing my vehicle across the highway as if it had been catapulted from a slingshot. The injuries I sustained from the collision instantly fragmented my life, creating a whirlwind of confusion and uprooting forty-one years of stability.

I was raised in a loving, stable, Christian home. My mother gave my brother and me the most precious gift any parent could give their child: a clear understanding of what it meant to have a personal relationship with Jesus Christ. She taught us the importance of placing Him first in our lives, as Lord. It was not until I became much older that I fully realized how difficult it must have been to raise two children alone. My mother depended heavily on God to provide every need, communing with Him daily for guidance. Hand in hand with that dependence was her spirit of determination to be proactive, blending God's guidance with her own commitment to uphold the responsibility He had given her.

I had witnessed firsthand His provision and faithfulness, in my mother's life as well as my own. I never experienced the void some children feel growing up without a father present. My mother's love and my Heavenly Father's continued presence reassured me throughout my impressionable tender years that I was carefully designed, formed, and worthy of the life I had been created for. I deeply loved my Heavenly Father and was secure in knowing I was His child.

I married at the gentle age of eighteen, and my life held endless opportunities. My husband Kip was my best friend, our individual families blended well together, and our two children blessed our lives beyond description. I was ever aware of the wonderful role model Kip fulfilled as a faithful husband and devoted father. Raising two precious children filled our lives with indescribable joy. Ever active, their growing years involved piano lessons, drum lessons, music festivals, choir concerts, band concerts, various sports activities and wonderful friendships. Kip and I were Sunday school teachers, children's club leaders, driving instructors and "puppy love" advisors. Kip was also a much-loved fishing guide for anyone who was interested, regardless of age!

Professionally, my career flourished. I worked in administrative positions for two well- established firms. One position involved organizing a staff of seven representatives who were directly accountable to a particular manager in a large insurance firm. Another position involved administrative work for ten engineers who were responsible for a large project within a productive oil company. Our decision to raise a family placed me into a role more satisfying than any other, the role of motherhood, which I retained until our youngest went to kindergarten.

Electing to move to the west coast opened the door to a new profession, enabling me to utilize many of my existing professional skills. I was hired as an assistant manager for a retail clothing outlet. A brand new store was opening in our community, so I travelled by ferry during the week to train at another store, returning home on weekends. Following completion of my training, the manager and I hired staff and got the retail outlet up and running.

Some years later, Kip opened his own business. In 1994, he invited me to join him, blending our skills as a professional team. Our love and friendship carried over to the professional area of our lives, deepening the special relationship we shared. Life seemed to be coasting along nicely before the accident. Our daughter married three months prior and our son was in his last year of high school. Our children now grown, Kip and I were looking forward to the "second honeymoon" stage, with all kinds of dreams and plans filling our heads.

In its uncertainty, however, life does not always flow without some kind of resistance or change in direction. Throughout our marriage, a few fairly significant difficulties managed to challenge, test and refine us as individuals, as a family and in our careers. At times it was as if a thin fog blurred our focus, making us question the pathway we were on. But we constantly relied on the Lord to see us through *any* situation. We sought His guidance and we sought the clarity that comes through trusting Him. Without fail He always provided.

However, the days, months and years following the car accident of November 7, 2001, were going to challenge us far beyond any struggle we had experienced. One single unexpected moment in time drastically altered my world as I had known it—*our* world as we had known it. Immediately following the accident, everything became scattered as if someone had cruelly tossed all the pieces of my life into the air, leaving them fragmented in a muddled heap. I didn't know where to start putting some of the pieces back together. I didn't know how. I couldn't really pinpoint what was wrong. The very core of my character, faith and personal self-worth felt as though it was shattered to pieces. I was really scared.

I invite you to share a small portion of my journey as I strive to reveal how God has held me, challenged me, sustained me, grown me and loved me through some of my darkest days. I have often bowed before the Lord God Almighty asking Him what my calling is *now*. What is His purpose for my life *now?* I've needed to carefully listen for His answer. I've pleaded for patience in my waiting as I hungrily sought His wisdom.

This book was His answer. Although I am sharing the traumatic event which has taken place in my life, my heart is powerfully aware of individual struggles, difficulties and challenges every human being encounters along this road of life. My deepest desire is to illuminate God's Word, God's faithfulness, and God's ever-present love to each reader. God Almighty is authentic. There is no second best. He is Alpha, the Beginning and He is Omega, the End. His love encompasses every human life and when we enter into a personal relationship with the Lord Jesus Christ, we have the divine privilege to freely access the very Creator of all. Anytime, anywhere.

I also wish to provide some kind of insight for those who have loved ones experiencing heartaches of any kind. Through understanding, compassion, encouragement, support, acceptance, and loads of patience, oceans of impossibilities and hopelessness can be transformed into mountains of possibilities, victories and hopefulness, rebuilding confidence that brings with it vibrant and healthy self-esteem. A hopefulness that reverberates with the realization, "I *am* worthy!" My writing is personal, as are my experiences. The first few chapters detail problems, challenges and difficulties which callously entered my world. I wish to share my journey from the very beginning, complete with the effects of my injuries as well as the impact they have had on my self-esteem. At the lowest point I found myself in a place of complete brokenness and confusion. Gratefully, through God's grace, tenderness and faithful love I did not remain in that deep dark cavern of grief.

Joy, strength, confidence and abundant life are the very reasons I needed to write this book. As you read the chapters revealing the root of my difficulties, please remember I am not simply "complaining" about all the things that have gone "wrong" since my accident. To remain cemented there would be a travesty, as the Light that shines ahead is worth focusing on and rejoicing over! Without sharing the personal side of my pain and difficulties, the incredible impact of God's power could perhaps seem trite and insignificant. After all, when life coasts along with only minor bumps we are able to cope with, it is easy to uplift and glorify the Lord. It is also easy to uplift ourselves. Yet through tough times of pain, emptiness and turmoil, God's love will blanket us entirely if we seek Him with a surrendered and open heart. Only then can we experience Him in a much deeper and personal way.

My efforts to be consistent and accurate are sincere, however due to the nature of my injuries the sequence of my writing may be somewhat disheveled, although I have spent endless hours trying to make them understandable and consistent. I have rummaged through personal journals to recapture certain events and emotions as they took place. I pray the following pages will bring honour and glory to the only One Who can truly provide abundance of life, our Heavenly Father. It is He Who gives life itself. He is the Faithful One Who reminds me moment by moment that yes, I am worthy.

Please join me.

PART ONE

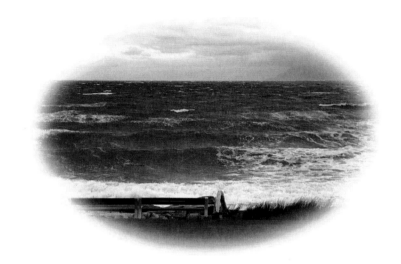

WHO IS THIS STRANGER?

"But when he asks, he must believe and not doubt,
because he who doubts is like a wave of the sea, blown
and tossed by the wind."
(James 1:6)

Photo © 2011 Kathleen M. Pritchard

1

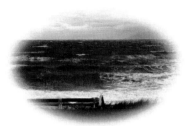

Waves of Uncertainty

Reflecting back to the days following the accident was difficult but very healthy for me. That one moment—on that particular day, at that particular time—changed the course of my life. I was unquestionably unprepared for the surge of emotions and challenges I was about to face.

Visible physical damage to my body was fairly minimal, although I will always experience some chronic pain. I knew the visible physical injuries could have been much more severe. Injuries to my neck, left shoulder, and lower back were going to require changes in how I did certain things. Any activity requiring me to raise my arms above my shoulders was pretty much taboo now, and lowering my head to write, sew, read, or paint caused severe muscle pain in my left shoulder area, resulting in tension headaches that often lasted three days. Keyboarding needed to be kept to a minimum, because of the positioning of my head and upper body. When in conversation, it was important for me to face the other person directly to avoid ensuing pain.

My husband Kip witnessed the entire accident as it transpired. The individual passed Kip's van at a treacherously high speed on a corner of the highway. He hadn't realized my van was stopped ahead, waiting to turn left off the highway. The impact was enormous.

Shortly after the accident, Kip explained what had happened. He had been driving a safe distance behind me and knew that I was going to turn off the highway at the next intersection. When the speeding car flew past him as he rounded the corner, he knew the driver wouldn't be able to stop in time. Terror gripped him as he had no recourse but to watch the collision take place. He had been frantic, knowing he was helpless to stop it. He kept praying I was still alive as he ran to my van amidst glass and pieces of my vehicle.

Personal recall of the days and months that followed is very sketchy, although bits and pieces have been disclosed to me as time passed. I experienced memory loss of what had taken place during various patches of time. However, I *was* aware that something was terribly wrong. I had extreme difficulty being in a room where music was playing or various people were in conversation. My attempts to administer familiar paperwork at our boutique were thwarted. Conversing with clients, friends, or family brought bouts of confusion, extreme fatigue, and nausea which often weakened me to the point of almost collapsing.

I would hear people speak, yet their words were scrambled, as if I was in a virtual game of Scrabble with the letters all mixed up and then flung toward me visually and audibly. Nothing made sense. I desperately tried to concentrate, to understand. Understanding avoided me. Multitasking was futile, resulting in constant frustration, as the familiarity of day-to-day activities was strangely foreign. Word-finding played hide-and-seek as my thoughts and lips didn't cooperate with one another. Confusion was rampant and endless questions flooded my head. I was afraid, very afraid.

I had to remind myself that God is *always* in control. He *could* have chosen to prevent the accident, commanding angels to divert the other car. He *could* have altered the timing slightly, or He *could* have taken me Home that afternoon. But He didn't do any of these. *Why? Why* did He allow this accident to take place and *why* did He allow my familiar life to become so foreign? I found myself strangely unsettled as I searched for explanations as to why I was so confused in familiar surroundings. Finding solutions to problems had always been my life's motto, but first I had to identify the problem itself.

Shopping, whether grocery shopping or otherwise, was extremely intimidating. As I entered a store, every single audio and visual presence encased me as though I was shoved into a kaleidoscope which was rotating at a tremendous speed, causing each colour and image to scramble into the next uncontrollably. I became disoriented, confused, nauseated, and lost. My memory often placed me in a state of emptiness as I drifted without direction. Stopping, I would try to *really* concentrate on what I needed to do and where I needed to go. Frustrated, I felt as though I was staring at an empty chalkboard, unable to access any information. Formerly effortless tasks, such as grocery shopping, now took many hours to accomplish and resulted in immeasurable fatigue. I would stare at my list only to find the words not registering. I found myself wandering from aisle to aisle in a grocery store where I had shopped for years.

Frustration grew and tears flowed as I would lie in bed at night, the events of the day racing through my mind mercilessly, replaying certain situations where understanding had evaded me. Restlessly, I tried to figure out what was causing such upheaval in my life, yet answers were beyond my reach. I desperately needed sleep to wash over me, my mind needing rest so I could find strength and energy for the following day.

Although I would often wake up somewhat tired, I still found myself eager to begin each brand new day. I secretly hoped I would experience marked signs of improvement. I felt encouraged by my anticipation of the events that would fill the day, but by midmorning I wrestled with the stark fact that my situation remained tumultuous and disorderly. I firmly believed that the foundation for overcoming anything was encapsulated within a positive attitude, yet questions relentlessly continued to mount as individual situations threw new, annoying curveballs at me. Answers remained absent.

Music held a special place in my heart. Having been musically inclined since I was a young teenager, music played a vital role in my life.

I was a member of my junior high and high school bands, the clarinet being my instrument of choice. I took piano lessons at the age of twelve and loved playing the piano tremendously. Singing in choirs brought incredible joy for many years, and for a brief period I enjoyed playing handbells at our church. Wherever I was, music was likely to fill the room, car, or boutique.

Kip also enjoyed music, having played the trumpet in his teen years. Our children grew up with music as a constant companion, its presence filling most of their waking hours at home. Following the accident, I instantly sought refuge in this musical harbour. To my dismay, anguish was the harbourmaster denying entry into the breakwater of this haven. I couldn't work, think, or correctly function when melodies started to flood my head, and flood they did. One note ran into another, then another, as if tripping over each other in succession.

Suddenly, the music which had brought such delight to my life converted into an incessant irritant as I tried to work, prepare meals, engage in conversation, or spend time shopping. I had counted on music to be of great solace for me as I focused on other, more pronounced areas of deficiencies. I experienced great sorrow over the loss of my ability to immerse myself in this musical sanctuary. I felt I had lost my place of peace, my harbour of renewal. *Why* this also, Lord? *Why?*

Always aware of God, I spoke to Him frequently—that's one thing that didn't change. But the simplicity of our chats changed dramatically. Ongoing questions were always on my lips and I began to vent frustration with my inadequacies. My prayers were messy and without substance as sentences got muddled up. Remaining focused and attentive during my prayer time was difficult, if not impossible. However, I eventually managed to state my wish list. I became extremely frustrated, because God wasn't miraculously making things clearer. I was trying to be patient but days, then months were passing by without any answers, nor any change. I became so focused on wanting answers that my time with God became half-hearted. I loved Him so much, yet I couldn't fathom why He was being silent to my pleas.

I was walking an unknown and completely unfamiliar path I did not want to be on. I was frightened and unable to foresee the road ahead.

Most daunting was the agonizing realization of the turmoil going on inside of me, shaking the foundation of my life on a daily basis, yet nothing on the outside visibly changed.

2

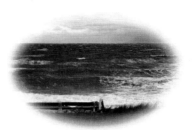

PERMANENT DISABILITY

PRIOR TO MY ACCIDENT, VISITS TO SEE OUR PHYSICIAN INVOLVED annual physicals, occasional illnesses with the kids and basic medical care. He had been our family physician for many years and I greatly respected him. Following the accident, I went to see him on a regular basis due to the struggles I was battling. He closely monitored my health and situation. Not being a physician who quickly jumps to conclusions without thorough investigation, he listened attentively to my concerns, and shared his professional advice with me and my husband. He was a trusted professional and I was grateful to him for allowing me to shed my tears and frustrations openly during a few rough periods.

Since I was often getting confused during my medical appointments, Kip attended with me. I referred to him as "my back-up brain." Crucial information I missed, Kip understood. Following the appointments, we would go to a park or sit in the car by the ocean. It was a quieter, more private time and place, and he would slowly explain to me what had been said. I *wanted* and *needed* to know what was happening within my body.

Kip's attendance to these medical visits turned out to be much more than valuable support and back-up. He brought to light situations I had either forgotten or not recognized. He also spoke guy language, which greatly simplified explanations at times. He told it exactly as he saw it. One phrase I do specifically remember was, "She's just not firing on all pistons." The explanation was immediately understood!

I was encouraged to be patient. Time was needed for healing to take place within my body, and only time would reveal certain answers. Ongoing medical observation revealed that my symptoms were the result of some type of trauma to the head and/or brain. It was crucial for me to acknowledge that time alone would determine the degree to which healing would take place and how much damage had occurred. That degree of healing was largely dependent on the extent of the injuries and area of the brain that was injured. If the symptoms continued, there was a high probability that some type of damage did exist, but *what* damage and to what degree?

As time passed, my physician expressed concern about the problems that were remaining persistent, with no sign of improvement. Having known me as a patient for many years, he had first-hand knowledge of the differences continuing to expose themselves since the accident. He knew more investigation was needed. During the next two years, a large part of our lives involved trips to medical professionals and specialists in neurology, psychology, neuropsychology, and head trauma. Kip had to accompany me on these trips as I was unable to drive at night, in the snow, in pelting rain, or in unfamiliar city traffic. I was also unable to adequately converse with others in busy situations. Living in a smaller oceanside community, our only highway to these appointments was by ferry—two ferries one direction to a main city and one ferry the other direction to another city. I have to admit, I was ill-prepared for the diagnosis that was concluded through extremely thorough testing. The early stages of testing initiated concern that I had acquired a Mild Traumatic Brain Injury. Further testing confirmed it.

I was devastated when I heard the term "Mild Traumatic Brain Injury." I did not understand exactly *what* that meant but knew well enough that the words "brain injury" weren't like being diagnosed with the flu. I knew what I was *living* through and what I had been living through since the accident. I *knew* it was not improving, although I tried optimistically to tell myself otherwise. However, I *never* anticipated the permanence of the injuries. I had remained focused on the hope that improvements would take place sometime down the road. If I just tried hard enough.

Neuropsychological testing was done, twice. Results from this intense form of testing revealed that the area of my brain responsible for processing information at a normal speed had been damaged. Along with the same conclusive results of other testing, answers were beginning to surface along with explanations as to *why* so many difficulties had arisen since the accident. All information going into my brain twenty-four hours a day, seven days a week, visually or audibly, was being processed much more slowly than normal. To me it felt as though the input of stimuli going through my brain for understanding was in slow-motion, while the noises and images themselves were in fast forward. An increase of activity during any situation greatly affected by my brain's ability to *process* the information, thwarting my ability to function normally.

One medical professional cleverly used a word picture to help Kip and me understand the process more clearly. He (somewhat teasingly) advised me that my brain really needed a "de-scrambler." He explained that new information was overlapping onto previous information too quickly when there was an overload of stimuli, causing mayhem with my brain's ability to take in, process, and relay the input at the speed it was going in. The messages ended up in a scrambled state, making no sense at all to me, disallowing me to function normally in life.

This constant overload was also responsible for the extreme fatigue I experienced, as the input along with continual, intense concentration was draining energy from my body. I spent valuable energy trying to cope with sensory overload triggered by any active situation, and my brain just wasn't able to keep up, my body following suit. When overwhelmed by excess stimuli resulting in extreme fatigue and nausea, grey spots blurred my vision, warning me to find a quiet place to rest *immediately* in order to avoid passing out.

Kip, my ever-faithful illustrator, was able to simply explain the cause and effect of my brain's function. We had some trouble one year with our motor home. After driving down to the base of a certain mountain pass through the Columbia Icefield, our motor home suddenly experienced complete power failure. No power brakes, no power steering, no power at all! Without warning, *every* function *immediately* shut down. Kip tried to safely maneuver this very large vehicle over to the side of the mountain highway. It was frightening.

We discovered that if we waited five or six hours and tried to start the vehicle again, the engine *would* crank over and we'd be fine for the next few hours. Once we got to a city (after being towed on a flat deck for five hours through the mountains), extensive diagnostic testing revealed that the computer module which transmits a message to the engine, telling it that there was adequate fuel flowing, failed. It kept shorting out after any long incline/decline passes. This was possibly due to extreme heat produced by one caliper, which had seized. Even though there was plenty of fuel in the tank, the computer module shorted out and we experienced total power failure. Everything shut down.

The demand on the vehicle to climb, then descend these mountain passes with a malfunctioning part likely caused it to short out, resulting in a complete loss of power. Once we had the computer module and our brakes replaced with new parts, our trips through these same passes were very relaxing and enjoyable. Instead of worrying about the vehicle itself, we were able to shift our focus toward experiencing the pleasure of the beauty around us.

Through this illustration, Kip helped me grasp a much clearer understanding of my brain injury. My brain, like the computer module, shorted out when too much demand was placed on it. There had been permanent damage to my brain, causing it to short out from sensory overload. Since the brain controls all other parts of the body's functions, this instantly shut down all of my energy reserve as well. Mental *and* physical power failure!

Unlike the malfunctioning computer module, my brain *would* send warning signs such as blurred vision, nausea and risk of blacking out. Kip has manually steered me up stairs or to a sofa when my legs would not carry me to a resting place. Also unlike the computer module in our motor home, my brain could not be disconnected and replaced with a brand new, perfectly functioning part. It became evident I needed to learn to work with what I had. I would have to pay very close attention to the warning signs that would indicate serious risk of personal power failure.

Memory problems, particularly with short-term memory, compounded my challenges. For the most part, long-term memory still had the ability for recall; however, segments of long-term memory sometimes failed me. Sporadic prompts initiated recall of certain people or activities such as names, faces and places, but I still had trouble clarifying various aspects of the event. On other occasions I could not bring to surface memories of particular incidences that had taken place in previous years. Drawing a blank really felt peculiar, especially when the recollection of that specific situation came so easily for others. Challenges with memory were quite variable and intermittent, and seemed especially dependent on many factors such as fatigue, familiarity, and mental visual recollection such as names I had written on file folder labels while operating our boutique.

One of the most innocent yet difficult questions for me to answer was, "What did you do today?" or "What do you have planned for the weekend?" I was unable to access the answer. My mind felt as empty as an untouched chalkboard. I *knew* my days were full, but I was often unable to pull up the information on the spot. Given half an hour or more, I would have been able to give an accurate answer.

Short-term memory loss was more of a continual challenge. This kind of memory loss can be as instantaneous as one moment ago or one hour ago. Everyone at some time experiences brief moments of forgetfulness. But, I was not simply forgetting something from time to time. Repeatedly I would do things that, one moment later, I had forgotten I had already done. I would pull milk out of the fridge, place it on the counter, then turn around and go back to the fridge to get milk.

Or, I would choose a top to wear for the day, lay it on the bed, then go back into the closet to decide what to wear.

One evening, I helped my husband pull back the sheets and comforter to get ready for bed. We then went into the washroom to brush our teeth. When I was finished, I walked back to our bedroom, ready to pull down the bed. I saw the sheets folded back and returned to the washroom to thank him for being so thoughtful. He looked somewhat bewildered, then gently reminded me that we had done that together. I looked blankly at him, trying to evoke that memory. It remained elusive.

This type of short-term memory loss was taking place quite often and was a little scary at first. Excellent memory had previously been part of my daily make-up. Kip used to call me his "walking dictionary," as I could easily recall almost anything. It is part of the reason we worked so well together. His strengths were design and consultations, while mine were administrative. It was an eerie feeling when I had just completed a task, yet the memory card in my head registered blank or fragmented as to what I had just done.

Word-finding was also a challenge, but not nearly so discouraging. It provided some humour when viewed as such. Many times, words spilled out of my mouth in a comical manner. Instead of saying, "I've got to go now," my words danced around like changing partners: "I've to got go now." I didn't realize this was even occurring until someone giggled at what I had said! Sometimes in mental replay, I could hear what I had said and found it a great opportunity to spontaneously chuckle.

During the first two years or so, I found myself hesitating before saying Kip's name. He had been my best friend since I was seventeen years old. We met at a youth group barbecue. During a baseball game, he was guarding first base. After I hit the ball (which was amazing in itself), I ran, then *slid* onto first base. He looked down at me and, with a heart-melting smile, said, "No one *slides* onto first base." I stood up, dusted myself off, and with a heart-melting smile of my own informed him that I do, and reminded him I was safe!

Our love affair was a hit from that moment on. Imagine the shock I felt when his name wouldn't just roll off my lips. I had to really think before feeling confident enough to say my own husband's name! When I did say it, I tried to replay it quickly inside my head to be sure I had said the right name. Fortunately, no other name tumbled out of my mouth!

Similar traits were being revealed in my writing as I found myself writing words in reverse order. Not always, but often enough to notice. When I first discovered this, I was appalled. The English language had always been a very strong point for me, and I couldn't believe I was mixing words up, verbally *and* on paper!

My method of reading was another interesting feature of this disability. Immediately following the accident, I found reading extremely difficult and did away with notions of settling down with a good novel. There was too much information to absorb and I had an enormously difficult time concentrating. However, through persistence and research I realized how important it was to continually feed and challenge my brain. I found myself able to read in short spurts, as long as paragraphs were of smaller proportions. Reading early in the day would reap the greatest benefit, as my attention span and energy levels depleted quickly from mid-afternoon on. Quite fascinating to me was the ensuing awareness of how I would pick up a magazine and automatically flip from back to front. Almost without fail I would go through magazines page by page beginning at the very *end* of the magazine, working my way toward the front.

Learning and applying new ways to do things or finding myself in an unfamiliar situation really tested my self-confidence. After moving into the home on my husband's family heritage property, I had a lot of new things to become familiar with. The home and property were familiar, which was an enormous blessing; however, some items previously *in* the home were not as familiar. The stove was one of them. I was endlessly turning on the wrong burner, leaving it exposed, having placed a pot on a different burner. I kept wondering why on earth food was taking so long to get warm! And, an exposed activated burner was dangerous (I found *that* out the hard way one day!). As much as I tried to train myself which knob belonged to which burner, I was having no success.

A wonderful tip passed on to me literally saved my bacon. The suggestion came from the Executive Director of the local Brain Injury

Group. She suggested I put coloured stickers on the compatible knobs and burners. I used green stickers (which said, "Great Job" with a happy face) to associate the front burner knobs with the front burners, and yellow stickers (which said, "You did it" with a happy face) for the back burners. The colours identified which knob to turn on, and the little messages were instant encouragement! (Even in writing this I had to mull over the wording many times to make certain I linked them up properly!)

Distinctive hearing problems were also difficult. Far different from an inability to hear, I was grappling with an unusually high sensitivity to noise. Noises like chainsaws, high pitches in various forms such as fans on refrigerators, dogs with repetitive barking (particularly high-pitched yapping), and piccolos increased the complexity of my situation. My head felt as though it would explode like a balloon filled with too much water. One morning at church, I had to slip out during a fiddle/cello duet. It was a lively piece and the fiddler was excellent. However, the pitch of the fiddle, along with the pace of the music, made it unbearable for me to stay in the sanctuary. Another Sunday, only the cellist played a piece and I was able to enjoy it immensely.

Any repetitive sound, such as the bass on a boom box or the incessant pounding of a hammer was agonizing. That really baffled me, as they do not have a high pitch. The beat just seemed to trip over itself as my brain tried to process each methodical sound. One beat seemed to echo several times, followed by the next beat, then the next. By the fourth or fifth beat, I was still processing the hollow echoes of the ones prior to it. I could only try to explain it this way: it sounded as if I were standing in the centre of a music room surrounded by an all-percussion band. One drummer would begin to practice, then a second drummer began a separate rhythm, until each drummer was warming up, and none of the rhythms were the same. The result? Chaotic noise! I found it impossible to carry on or understand a conversation when audio activity rampantly flooded my head.

The initiation of the first three years seemed to go by ever so slowly. Questions, fear, testing, trials, information, answers and insight swept Kip and me through a torrent of confusion and unknowns, finally bringing us to a place of definition. I was conclusively diagnosed as having a Mild Traumatic Brain Injury; the *source* of what was causing such upheaval within my body was finally identified. This intruder now had a name.

The rest of life was ahead of me, and although I could label the culprit, I still had to figure out what to do in order to cope with the changes. I needed to figure out how to progress in light of the losses that had occurred. I felt great uncertainty, because I still had no idea what to expect from one day to the next. There was so much I wasn't prepared for. Life itself would continue to give me daily lessons.

PART TWO

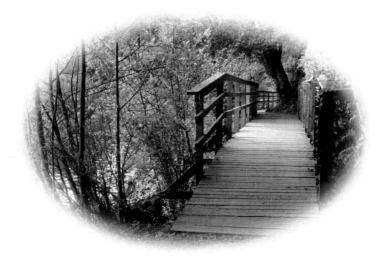

JOURNEY OF DISCOVERY

"Your word is a lamp to my feet and a light for my path."
(Psalm 119:105)

1

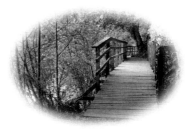

Lifelong Transitions

We are blessed to live on one of the prettiest beaches I've ever seen. Kip's grandparents have owned property in this bay since 1935, and he and his family have spent countless years of enjoyment on this beach. Kip and I are both very honoured to continue this family heritage, being the third generation to call this property home. Our long-term goal is to restore much of it back to its original state.

We moved to this property in the fall of 2004, three years after my accident. Kip and I found great repose in the rush of the wind through the enormous fir trees, and in the power of the surging waves during that first wintry season living on the beachfront. It was a wonderful haven away from the restless world of busyness.

Spring brought with it a special beauty that can only be found on the coast. It was a glorious introduction to the warm months of summer. I was introduced to this beautiful spot shortly after we were married. Its immense beauty and rich heritage quickly claimed a place of its own within my heart, and as our family grew, our children spent their summers playing on this coveted beach. The long-awaited warm days generated an abundance of outdoor activities and our beach came to life with families, children and dogs. Ah, the sounds of summer! Aaaah! The sounds of summer! *Much* different from the solace of fall and winter, the arrival of the first summer living on the beachfront took the wind right out of my sails. I had forgotten how active and popular this particular beach could get. Or perhaps I hadn't forgotten—perhaps I hadn't noticed the flurry of activity before because I was involved with it just like everyone else, without the handicap of a brain injury.

Some days, more than one hundred people (and their barking "best friends") enjoy the stretch of sand in front of our home. I realize that to many folks reading this, having one hundred people out on the beach may seem like a very minute number. Most cities with beaches have thousands of people claiming every little space of sand. Yet with my brain injury, one hundred people were as overwhelming as one-hundred thousand. I had been looking forward to this season a lot, not at all aware of what lay ahead. I had not travelled this road of brain injury before, and normal situations cruelly brought challenges I could not foresee or prepare for. I didn't know that this particular problem existed until I found myself smack-dab in the middle of it. Despite understanding the cause of my struggles and limitations, I was not prepared at all for this distinctive set of difficulties, nor the emotional turmoil that would ripple endlessly throughout the longer, sun-drenched days.

During the three years immediately following my car accident, I had been able to retreat to our previous home up the road to find relief from the abundance of activity down on the beach. Having been able to previously slip away at times of overload, I was unprepared for the toll it would take not having anywhere to escape to. June brought the first discovery of what would become the norm for the duration of the summer. While at the kitchen window one day, I noticed movement out of the side of my eye. Staring down the beach, my eyes almost popped out from their sockets! A steady stream of children from a rural school were marching toward our home frontage, anticipating a wonderful day at the beach. Instantly I was reminded of the song, "The ants go marching one by one, hurrah, hurrah…" I glanced the other direction. Cars and trucks had lined up along our fence, and parent volunteers were spilling out of them. Quickly, shade tents and coolers brimming with food and drinks for the day took their ceremonial place on the sand, right in front of our home!

I was delighted to see the excitement in the body language of the children. I absolutely adore children, and had been actively involved in our children's lives. I had also cared for infants ages zero to three in a childcare centre (along with two other caregivers) for a brief two-year period. Children and the beach seem to go together like peanut butter and jelly. They bring life to it, creating sandcastles, burying friends under the sand, and squealing with delight as the cool water sends chills throughout their bodies when they first get wet. Treasure hunts abound as eyes and bodies seek for crabs, sand-dollars, starfish and anything else that can only reside in this enchanting place. Not to mention the hours of work put into building magnificent forts created by endless imaginations and countless pieces of driftwood.

It was a beautiful day, and I had most of the beach-side windows open. I became absorbed in the delight of watching the scenes outside, losing myself in the excitement oozing from the children. Abruptly, however, the callousness of my brain injury allowed no room for selective gratification. To my disheartening surprise, I found myself wandering through the house, unable to concentrate or accomplish the tasks at hand. Extreme fatigue began to drain all energy from my body. I felt as though I was in a room filled with strangers who were all yelling at once in a foreign language. The high pitches that accompanied numerous squeals of delight were torturous to absorb. The sounds from the beach below were magnified as they were carried by the breeze up into every room of our home. With tears streaming down my face, I reluctantly and weakly closed every door and window. How could this be?

It was sensory overload in a massive overdose. I was thrown backward emotionally as I tried to grapple with this hideous intruder that seemed to threaten any part of goodness and joy that crossed my path. I was definitely unprepared for this jolt of cruelty that instantly encroached upon my entire being. I absolutely adored children, and was beside myself with sorrow over the realization that this disability was further depriving me of something else I cherished very deeply. I was desperate to unearth answers that would help me cope with this new stranger in my life and I ached to find help so I could retrieve the treasures of daily living that were mercilessly remaining obscure.

During an appointment with one particular specialist, I asked if I could do anything that may lessen the effects of the disability or help me overcome certain aspects of these difficulties. I asked how I could claim back some of my former capabilities. I wanted answers that would help me recoup my losses. This fellow was a psychiatrist who specialized in head trauma cases, and he wasn't going to mince words. We were told to envision someone who lost a leg. The harsh fact that the leg would never grow back again was undisputed. It could not be massaged, exercised, or strengthened, ever again. It was gone. Permanently.

Elaborating on the example of the lost leg, he told me that I *would not* be able to retrain my brain to perform as it used to. My brain would need to retrain *me* to do things differently. Choices and options for daily life would be determined by signals that I would need to recognize and become closely acquainted with. Signals I would *need* to respond to. Signals which would forever produce uncertainty, moment by moment, day by day, year to year.

He then informed me that the adaptations I was making were really good, but I would never move forward successfully again in life until I learned to accept my disability. I had responded somewhat audaciously, feeling confident that I had been learning to accept my brain injury and newly acquired disability quite well. I had worked very hard at trying to maintain a positive attitude, and I had made valiant efforts at trying to find solutions to the unwelcome but persistent limitations. What I really wanted to hear from him was a reply of optimism that this disability could be minimized, managed down to a simple annoyance. I didn't realize it, but I had wanted him to *say* what I was trying to *do*—sugar coat it.

"No," was the harsh, elevated reply, "You are *not* accepting it!" He told me firmly that I must accept the reality of having a permanent brain injury which was going to demand constant, life-long changes.

I was told that I must accept that I cannot will the brain injury to go away, and that my wishes for normality to return would be futile. He warned me not to dismiss the losses I was encountering, expecting them to return someday. He cautioned me about the danger of closing my eyes and my heart to the impact those losses were having on me and would continue to have on me. This was how it was going to be for the long haul. The only success I would find would be in my willingness to fully accept my disability. Success or failure would be heavily dependent on my willingness to acknowledge and respond to the signals, wholly accepting my limitations. The key element for success would be adhering to them.

This specialist was not unkind or cruel. He told it like it was and wanted to make sure Kip and I were armed with as much information as possible. The road ahead was going to challenge us, and he wanted us to be as prepared as we could be. Undeniably, tears flowed readily. Yet this man knew that we must face my disability head on. If we buried our heads in the quicksand of false hope, it would destroy not only me, but both of us.

Often referred to as the Invisible Disability, my type of injury rarely offers tangible or obvious clues. This fact created one of the most challenging aspects for unconditional acceptance. Out of sight, out of mind had a personal meaning attached to it. Because my disability was out of sight, there was a tendency to keep it out of mind, as in the case of my exuberance over the children spending the day down at our beach. I had forgotten all about my disability for those brief moments, because the routine that had begun to settle in throughout the fall and winter was becoming more familiar and my surroundings were fairly stable and self-monitored. When the sudden excess stimulation showed up, I did not recognize the signals and I did not understand what was taking place. I just knew the joy I felt had quickly reverted to tears, frustration and uncertainty. I was grieving and didn't even know it.

Acceptance is a journey of time, but I was encouraged that it would come if I allowed it. I was reassured that I would gradually become more accustomed to my limitations as we discovered and developed realistic boundaries. Those boundaries would need to be faithfully honoured.

Healthy acceptance of these limits and boundaries would be crucial to my progress and well-being. I needed to fully *accept* my disability and work with it, no sugar-coating added. Challenges will always arise, because every moment in life provides opportunity for unknowns. Even in the most normal and uneventful life, there is not one moment or plan in which absolute certainty is guaranteed. In view of the fact that my brain injury is unseen, invisible and unpredictable, the seriousness of my limitations can be very hard to understand and/or accept. For myself as well as others.

Three years of appointments with various specialists and medical professionals had unanimously confirmed the nature of my injury. All had concluded that a Mild Traumatic Brain Injury had taken up residence in my head and unfortunately there was no recourse to evict it! There were no set expectations as to what may or may not take place as the years progress, although there are certain phases that will have the potential to find common ground as time evolves. Medical forecasts predicted that the aging process may be more pronounced as a result of the brain injury. My disability would often place me in a cerebral position similar to someone in their eighties. The reduced ability to process information quickly would manifest itself in slower movements, delayed verbal responses, some short-term memory loss and decision-making struggles.

Lack of concentration became a constant. This area of deficiency really rattled me at first because I had possessed excellent focus all my life. Long-term plans became almost non-existent as my brain could only relate to what was taking place at the present time. Attempting to look beyond the day at hand or the day(s) to follow resulted in frustration and a sense of overload. I could not seem to grasp or retain much beyond the present. Thus, the reason I was not able to readily respond to the simple question, "What do you have planned for the weekend?"

Kip and I did make plans together and I became heavily dependent on the aid of a desktop calendar and palm pilot. I was encountering intermittent short-term memory loss and confusion when things went too quickly, and I found myself wandering unfocused at times, especially when I was very tired or in a busy place.

Some specialists informed me that the brain injury may present a higher risk factor for the onset of symptoms of Alzheimer's disease or other forms of dementia, should I already be a candidate for these diseases *without* the presence of the brain injury. In other words, if my normal future held the health risk of Alzheimer's or any other form of dementia, the potential was there to experience the symptoms of these diseases earlier than I normally would, perhaps with more pronounced difficulties.

Medically, there have been varying views on this particular prognosis, yet all professionals were in agreement that the brain injury would not initiate dementia. I wanted, and needed, to make sure I clearly understood what was being said. My understanding was that the brain injury would not cause the onset of dementia or Alzheimer's. The disease itself is a separate health issue. However, there is a possibility that the brain injury may magnify the symptoms of the disease, should the risk of it already be present within my body.

Our first introduction to this possibility was frightening for Kip and me, as we both were well aware of the struggles I was already dealing with. Once again, the health professionals and specialists were extremely helpful in educating us. They were committed to arming us with facts and legitimate possibilities so we didn't head into the future blind-sighted. Their assessments did agree that my brain injury would often expose areas of deficiency with the likelihood that those deficiencies will become more noticeable as the years progress and the natural aging process takes place. It may seem odd, but I found great comfort in the fact that I didn't know for certain what lay ahead. In actuality, nobody really, indisputably could know. Except the One Who made us.

I was finally receiving answers to the turmoil that had endlessly brought disorder to my life since the car accident. There were conclusive medical reasons for the vast changes that had shattered my previously comfortable and familiar world. The diagnosis and explanations, harsh as they seemed at times, launched a new and deeper understanding of my condition, allowing me and my husband to finally grasp what had been taking place and *why*.

The process of discovery was extremely difficult, but without going through it, Kip and I may have remained lost in a churning, confusing life which held no answers. Misdiagnosis may have taken place down the road had my brain injury not been correctly identified after a long and strenuous time of professional medical monitoring. Medical assessments enlightened Kip and me as to why I could not listen to music while being involved with another task, no matter how minimal. We were finally able to figure out why I couldn't drive under certain conditions and why decision-making took such a long time. Awareness started to unravel the whirl of questions that had held our world captive for so long. A whole host of whys were becoming much less frightening.

During a period when I was having a *lot* of testing done, my physician made a comment to me before leaving the examination room. He said with a smile, "By the way, Kathie, you *are* still smart!" Wow, that was music to my ears! How I appreciated that jewel of information, because I wondered at times if I was going crazy, or if I had become "slow." I knew I could still accomplish many important tasks; however, the time it took to accomplish them was multiplied by at least a factor of three. It was encouraging to hear that my level of reasoning and intelligence was still fully intact. As the testing progressed, I began to understand that my brain was reacting slower when trying to process the stimuli it encountered. Yet when speed was not an issue, and a quiet place was available, I was still able to achieve a healthy understanding.

I had observed something similar with Kip's father. He was diagnosed with Parkinson's disease in the 90s, and the disease, compounded by MSA (Multiple System Atrophy), damaged his physical body very quickly. He went Home to be with his Lord February 19, 2002, just three-and-a-half months after my car accident.

What I witnessed in this intelligent man's life remained with me and it often spurred me on to challenge my own limitations, within reason, remaining focused on what is ahead. Although his physical body was failing him, Kip's father's intelligence and wits were not impaired. He was exceptionally sharp-minded and brilliant. I found his quick sense of humour refreshing, despite the devastation to his body. The disease quickly robbed him of physical strength, eventually causing the muscles in his mouth to move much more slowly, and with great difficulty. When asked a question, he would take a considerable amount of time to reply.

It wasn't that he didn't know the answers. He most certainly did. He just couldn't make the answer come out quickly or clearly. Sometimes, folks would then address Kip's mother to retrieve the answer. This must have frustrated Kip's father enormously. He *could* answer and was capable intellectually of spinning circles around anyone who wished to chat with him. Yet many people didn't understand or weren't aware that all he needed was adequate time to respond.

I cherish deeply the last words he spoke to me. I pray I will never forget them. I had knelt down beside him, bidding him goodnight as he sat in his electric scooter. It was hard for him to raise his head to look up at people, so I often knelt to make it easier. His voice was also quite weak at that time. He slowly reached across his lap and placed his right hand on top of mine. Gently patting my hand and looking me square in the eye, he said, "Remember to take care of yourself." He passed away at home two days later.

I do not have a debilitating disease such as Kip's father had. However, I have been witness to the courageous spirit and strength that can radiate from within a person's being, despite health-related obstacles. I do know personally, to some degree, the frustration he must have felt not being able to quickly respond verbally when he was addressed. Inside of his head, and factually, he was still the brilliant, intelligent engineer who had been highly respected in his profession for decades. He was still the loving, kind and faithful husband, father and grandfather who had guided his family well. But his body was no longer strong. It had become frail. Yet his spirit, intellect and devotion resonated from deep within his soul.

Through his example and love, I often found myself contemplating those last words, "Remember to take care of yourself." It wasn't until sometime later I realized he was one of very few who could truly understand the challenges and frustrations I was encountering. His were much more pronounced because of Parkinson's disease, but to some degree I knew he understood. I believe he recognized the changes I was experiencing immediately after the accident. He knew I was smart, he knew I was hurting, and he wanted me to know the enormous importance of taking care of myself in order to achieve fullness of life despite the obstacles. Courageous yet tender advice, lovingly administered through a gentle pat on my hand and earnest eye-to-eye contact. I will always cherish the gift he gave me in that defining moment.

I was so grateful to have been medically educated during those first three years on the cause and effect of what was categorically diagnosed as a permanent disability. I was also encouraged by the support I was receiving from that team of medical professionals. I began to understand the importance and value of certain medications. Through careful investigation, specific medications were prescribed. These medications varied according to tolerance and effectiveness, so consistent monitoring was, and always would be, essential. Achieving levels of constancy continued to present a challenge as some medications worked favourably, while others did not. I was aware that different stages of my life would require adjustments in medication, but I had begun to view that as a good thing. Once stabilized, results were positive. When properly administered, medication can make an enormous difference in one's quality of life.

Additional nameless challenges continue to present themselves daily without warning, even with the aid of medication. That had been difficult to digest along with dashed hopes of being able to return to the lifestyle I once lived effortlessly, however I was perpetually encouraged to accept the permanence of the injury and to surrender myself to the inevitable *certainty* of uncertainty. Transitional stages would endure lifelong. How I responded to them was a choice only I could make. I could live a full life *with* the disability, discovering new horizons no matter how challenging, or I could just exist, succumbing to the limitations of the disability. I have always tried to be optimistic, and this reflection ignited a fire of renewed anticipation in me. I could still choose to find hope, to discover fullness in life once again. The option was there for the taking. The road before me was still very blurred and a little scary, but I wasn't going to turn my back on it.

I had been blessed with an abundance of information during those three years. I was now armed with knowledge as to what had happened to my body as a result of the accident, and I had been amply supplied with encouragement and guidelines on how to work *with* it. Several medical professionals were committed to supporting my efforts to move forward. A lot of uncertainties remained, but I felt as though I was no longer looking into a deep black hole of unanswered questions. I felt more prepared and confident to grasp the handle of the door that would reveal the first altered steps of my future.

I believe it's extremely important to be proactive. I wanted to make the most of my existing capabilities, of which there were many to still tap into. It was at this intersection that I prayerfully turned my focus toward seeking God's purpose for this life He obviously felt was worthy to still do His work. I was beginning to recognize His graciousness and love as He provided answers to Kip and me through outstanding medical professionals who patiently guided us toward a place of some understanding as we wrestled with a very complicated and invisible disability.

Eager to move forward, I needed time alone with God. Realistically, not pessimistically, I knew the road ahead was going to be filled with obstacles, challenges, failures and frustrations that would threaten to break me. Yet I strongly believed that new horizons of endless opportunities also awaited. Forging toward a healthy future would open doors of growth and renewed confidence. I felt more focused and eager to take those first steps, but I was also somewhat apprehensive, as I knew I was entering into a world where everything was completely different. The tests were done, the diagnosis given, the changes evident. Now it was my responsibility to take hold of the baton to do what only I alone could do. Success would be determined by my outlook, particularly through the rougher times.

Knowledge, understanding and acceptance are valuable tools when applied correctly, but they don't guarantee ease or continual success. I was opting to approach life from a completely foreign angle to overcome the succession of frustrations that played freely with my emotions since I had acquired my brain injury. I had tasted the turmoil of unwanted change through those extremely difficult years, and I was very aware of the futility in trying to move forward without placing my hand, my complete trust, and my very life into the divine care of the One Who created me.

The problem had been identified, and there was a stirring within my spirit to pursue concrete solutions. The time had come to straighten and polish the Armour of God. I was going to rely on it heavily as I advanced forward.

2

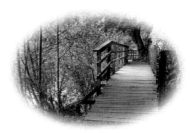

ALONE WITH GOD

I COMMITTED THREE FULL DAYS TO COMMUNING WITH MY HEAVENLY Father. This was something I needed to do alone. Although Christians share a special bond with each other because of our mutual faith, our relationship with Christ Himself must be personal. My husband is my very best friend this side of heaven. Our walk with the Lord is the foundation of our marriage. But there are intervals when it is critical to experience time alone with God, One on one. Communing privately with Him in complete stillness allows us to really know Him. Often during this time of intimacy we can hear Him speak to our hearts. Reserving time alone with God reveals the value you place on your personal relationship with Him. It is the very essence of what makes the relationship personal.

I turned to the sanctuary of our home. I could control the environment, ensuring it was what I needed it to be. I knew I would require frequent rests. I answered no phone calls, nor visits to the door. I saw my husband only in the early morning and evenings when he came home from work. Other than my contact with him, I vowed to shut myself off from the rest of the world to seek only God's Presence. This was not withdrawal. Rather it was a venue for spiritual renewal.

Jeremiah 29:13 says, *"You will seek me **and find me** when you seek me with **all** your heart"* (emphasis mine). St. Anselm of Canterbury beautifully captured the importance of intimacy with the Father when he wrote, "Enter into the inner chamber of your mind. Shut out all things save God and whatever may aid you in seeking God; and having barred the door of your chamber, seek Him." I wanted nothing to infringe on our time of communion. I greatly needed to spend time alone with my Father. I cannot begin to explain the shifting of emotions I experienced during this intimate time. Bowing before Him, I invited Him to draw near, cherishing my time in uninterrupted prayer. Subsequently, I asked Him for the courage to dig deep inside of myself to expose questions that were submerged in my troubled heart. I asked Him to blanket me with His peace as I went through this extremely difficult and vulnerable process.

Human wisdom had unlocked the door of medical mystery, yet knowledge of my disability was but a baby step forward. Knowledge is wasted if not applied. Applying all the necessary ingredients to confidently advance was going to take a lot of time and enormous patience. I had placed my grasp on the handle of the door leading to my future. Now I needed to fling it wide open to take hold of the powerful hand of my Heavenly Father, Who waited eagerly to guide me along the pathway of the unknown. Choosing a comfortable, bright room, my only resources consisted of blank paper, a couple of pencils and God's Word, the Holy Bible.

After spending considerable time in prayer I began to write down questions. Very slowly, at first. I asked God to lead me, to help me sort through the feelings that I needed to. I had so many questions, but I was having trouble sorting through them for the really important ones. I discovered that God wanted me to become fully aware of the fact that all of the questions were important to ask. There were no unimportant ones. I needed to surrender whatever lay within my soul in totality. Revealing my heart while searching for God's heart was life-changing.

Initially I found myself angry. I was surprised by this because I knew I was in God's Presence and had asked Him to be with me. Would He perhaps be angry with me for unleashing this deeply hidden emotion? Writing questions down, then pondering each one, made feelings surface I thought I had been handling, and hiding really well. After venting my anger, frustration and fears, tears softly began to flow. I believe it was the first time since the accident I really allowed myself to work through emotions I had tried to toughen up against. I'm certain I added immeasurably to the ocean's abundance that initial day of candid soul-searching.

I had worked very hard to give the outward appearance of being strong, to let others know as well as myself that I was okay with what had happened to me. I would smile and put on a superficial mask as though this was something I could handle and "work through." After all, I knew God would never give me more than I could bear. I had refused to really face the truth regarding the strain the disability was placing on me, hoping the unwanted changes would slowly disappear, despite the warnings as to the importance of a spirit of acceptance.

Although tears had privately flowed at times because of frustration over my inability to do something, I had never truly allowed myself to grieve the loss of who I had been. I didn't know at that time what it really meant to grieve my losses. My heart ached, craving to be restored to the old me. Catching glimpses of my unmarked frame in the mirror, I occasionally chastised myself for acknowledging those emotions. Visibly, I was the old me, so why was this inward battle taking place? Why did I still feel so foreign in this familiar body, even though I knew medically what was wrong with my brain?

The emphasized words of one specialist kept surfacing: "No, you are *not* accepting it." Mulling that sentence over, scrutinizing it to lay bare the importance of the words, I finally began to explore more deeply what he had meant, not just what he said. The more I pushed, fought against, and resisted the limitations of my disability, the more I robbed myself and others of the acceptance of my disability. This word *acceptance* was an enormous hindrance I would encounter time and time again. I knew the only way to have victory in the acceptance of my disability was to seek the Father's guidance and strength. Obviously, I hadn't been able to achieve that on my own.

Sharing the very core of my heartaches with my Father during those three days allowed me to be angry, scared, vulnerable and exposed before Him. He listened to my doubts and fears, and He openly allowed me to lay it all on the line without intervention. He faithfully listened without harsh judgment or criticism. I was free to say whatever was on my heart in complete candour.

Opening His Word and becoming immersed in my time with Him instilled personal recognition of how His love heals an utterly broken heart. God's Word, the Holy Bible, enables Him to speak to our hearts when we truly seek to hear Him. So does prayer. Sharing in simple and honest communion, He began to ask me some difficult questions. Did I doubt Him? Did I question His purpose for my life? Did I feel less of a person because of the limitations that had become part of my daily life? Was I really worth any less because my life changed course in an instant?

Alone with Him, I was lovingly reminded that He has known from the beginning of time what course my life would take. His personal unconditional love for me, His precious child, is the very reason I have life! God's divine promise to be faithful far surpasses any promises made by another human being, even with the best of intentions. He encouraged me to remember my life was not ended that day, just re-directed to a different pathway. Would I trust Him? Would I be willing to submissively accept what He had allowed?

God promised to remain by my side just as He always has. He promised to help, guide and strengthen me. He has promised His unconditional love with accessibility to Him twenty-four hours a day, seven days a week. No appointment necessary. When I want to speak with Him, He has vowed to be present and faithful. What then was my responsibility? What did He want me to do? Opening His Word, I read Psalm 9:9–10: *"The LORD is a refuge for the oppressed, a stronghold in times of trouble. **Those who know your name will trust in you, for you, LORD, have never forsaken those who seek you"** (emphasis mine). His response was clear. I was counselled to place unwavering trust in Him, believing beyond any doubt that He is more than faithful in upholding that trust.

It was time for spiritual cleansing and renewal. It was time to ask for God's forgiveness. It was time to seek God's will and purpose for my life. This meant surrendering my own will, my denial, and my life, exactly as it was, completely to Him. The choice to set aside those three days, seeking God and finding Him, allowed me to turn the handle on the door of my future. Now, the door was open and willingly I reached out to feel the Master's hand firmly clasp mine. I knew the road ahead was going to bring surprises and challenges. I knew the road would be bumpy. Placing my trust in God didn't mean all the problems, challenges and difficulties were going to be eliminated. I knew my disability was permanent and its effects would last a lifetime.

But now my perspective had changed. God had made some serious alterations inside of my heart. My willingness to place complete trust in God Almighty ensured I would not walk this journey alone in the fog of uncertainty and doubt with apprehension and trepidation nipping at my heels. God reached down to the very core of my being and cleansed me. He renewed my spirit, and my heart was like a fresh, clean canvas, ready and waiting for the Master's touch.

Spending this time alone with my Heavenly Father permitted such freedom through uninhibited interaction. I was greatly encouraged and more focused on what needed to be done. Best of all, I was still Kathie, the one whom God had created. I was loved very deeply and I was loved unconditionally. I rolled up my sleeves, optimistic and ready to get started on this new pathway. My medical questions had been addressed, revealing an injury that would create challenges in my daily life permanently. Medical counsel had confronted my superficial interpretation of acceptance, forcing me to deal with the tangible effects of this brain injury pragmatically. And my loving God had waited patiently for me to seek Him out with an open heart, and a readiness to yield to His will.

The next few chapters walk through an important part of my journey. Although I had surrendered to God's leading and guidance, depending on Him for daily strength, I still had crucial lessons to learn. Emotions simply cannot be turned on or off at will. Stress greatly compounds and heightens the emotional side of a brain-injured person. When situations arise that are stressful and complicated, it is easy to become muddled and frustrated as workable solutions are not readily accessible.

Difficult to share, the following chapters reveal the emotional turmoil that invaded my world, even as I strived to remain close to the Lord. Satan, the master of cruelty, will intensify his attacks when we draw closer to God. He will tug, pull, yank, deceive and taunt even the most faithful follower of Christ. Satan can be very sly, and feelings of uncertainty can turn into powerful internal battles if he is allowed any room to work at all. Therefore, one must make a conscious and courageous decision to slam the door in his face, unmistakably declaring who is Lord.

I pray the following chapters will reveal how God can work in us and through us, enabling us to overcome any situation or circumstance. God wants us to trust Him, depend on Him and call upon Him, exchanging overwhelming feelings of defeat for an awareness of accomplishment, victory and priceless self-worth. Surrender to Him will be life-changing.

PART THREE

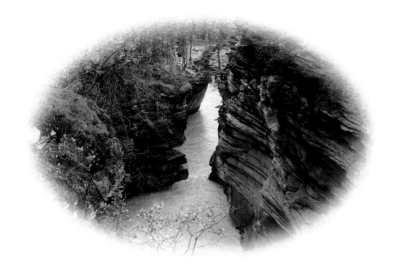

VALLEY OF EMOTIONAL TURMOIL

*"The LORD is close to the brokenhearted
and saves those who are crushed in spirit."*
(Psalm 34:18)

Photo © 2005 Kathleen M. Pritchard

1

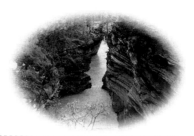

Battling Guilt

My entire life I had relied on my strong spirit to help me through certain trials, yet now my inner strength felt as though it was being tested beyond what I could endure. Knowledge and understanding of my disability was invaluable and a very important starting point, but it certainly didn't end all frustration. The continual process of learning how to adjust to my limitations didn't guarantee easy acceptance. Many times I felt I was battling an unseen adversary who was making me feel very inadequate. I was painfully aware of my recurring inability to accomplish what I viewed as the simplest of tasks. All too often, I found myself struggling with feelings of incompetence. Tears flowed readily and I would cry out to God, and to Kip, bewildered and frustrated by my perceived failures.

Socializing had been a very large part of our lives. People are such wonderful, intriguing creatures. I delighted in the joy of embracing new friends, yet also cherished the bond of long-established friendships. Social events constantly beckoned us and our family thrived as friendships were nurtured through enjoyable times of entertaining. Following the accident, however, interaction with others was draining every ounce from me, particularly in the evenings when social gatherings usually take place. Special occasions that once filled our home with laughter and joy were measurably reduced, and though I would attempt to entertain during certain holidays, my previous abilities just simply were not there. Fatigue engulfed me, making offers for dinner in our home scarce.

I had once soaked in the joy of fellowship with others, but due to the impact of one accident, my understanding of what was being said was lost. Laughter would erupt. I would attempt a smile, not knowing what the laughter was about. Plans were made, love was exchanged, joys and sorrows were shared. I watched people's mouths move and I saw smiles lighten their faces. Other times, I witnessed concern casting a shadow. I felt like an outsider watching through a windowpane without being able to mingle or understand what was taking place in the lives of those I love. I grieved deeply over this loss. I knew I was losing out on an enormous part of life. I would sit down with Kip during a quiet moment the day after and ask him questions about what had taken place. It felt as though a complete stranger inhabited my body and I didn't know what to do about it. My heart was aching to retrieve the simplicity of interacting with others who filled my life with so much joy. Very few people really knew the depth of helplessness and loss I felt not being able to participate in or understand conversations that occurred with familiar normality.

Kip and I discussed this issue a lot, and together we concentrated on searching for positive, workable adaptations. We had to, in order to move forward in our lives and in our marriage. We were committed to facing each obstacle and difficulty with complete faith that God would help us find effective solutions. Kip patiently stood right beside me. He encouraged me, lifted me up verbally (and physically at times), and took over many responsibilities at home. His display and words of love carried me through many difficult times despite the toll it was taking on him.

Kip became incredibly tired trying to run our business, find replacement staff, and manage a lot of tasks at home. He drove me to numerous doctor and specialist appointments, many out of town. Two ferry trips were generally required for each appointment, resulting in three-day absences from our boutique to allow for travel time and my health restrictions. Never once did he complain about or resent the time spent away from the boutique.

I was extremely concerned over the time lost at the boutique, very much aware of the fact that our income was at risk. He continually reassured me of God's faithfulness, reminding me that He had always taken care of us and would continue to do so. Weathering our share of storms, we have always relied on our Heavenly Father and each other. All that really mattered to Kip was that I was alive. I don't think anyone truly recognized the immense load he carried, and I was deeply concerned about him. Feelings of guilt seemed to constantly wash over me. I felt guilty about letting my husband down, letting my business partner down, letting my family down, letting friends down, and letting myself down. Why did I always feel so guilty when I was trying to do everything possible to reclaim some of my familiar life?

My ability to do things quickly was completely gone, as I needed to carefully think things through in order to accomplish something. This resulted in taking three times longer to do just one task. I'd say "sure" to doing something for someone only to discover that it was too difficult to do because of surrounding circumstances, or it was going to take too long to accomplish within their specified time requirement. I found myself not being able to complete the required task, and became discouraged because I had let someone down.

Denial of the reality of my limited abilities was a major stumbling block, and that denial was becoming an enemy I could not escape. My self-confidence began to decline as personal unrealistic expectations continually challenged my determination to accept the new me. I did not like that term, the new me. I wanted the old me back again, or at least some resemblance of who I had been. I felt irritated about my disability and the way it changed me.

My patience with these changes was heavily challenged. I found I became increasingly focused on my short-comings, deeply craving to feel whole again. I searched the depths of my soul to find ways to fully participate in life again, trying to tuck away any sign of my disability. When I fell short, I blamed myself for being incompetent. I saw failure. I felt I was a failure. That line of thinking was unrealistic, as my brain injury was responsible for imposing my disability, not my spirit. I believe I subconsciously expected God to supernaturally bring about success as I tried to grab hold of familiar and identifiable traits.

These were the lowest points in the stages of recovery as I endeavored to move forward with my life. Months passed by and I was confronted with the ruthless fact that there would be no full recovery of life as it had been. Admittedly, God had not told me there would be. He had promised to walk with me, yes, but He had never promised tangible, physical improvement. I could, and did, make adaptations. Great adaptations. Yet I would still push myself to limits that brought on two or three days of absolute exhaustion and fatigue afterward. Instead of feeling exuberant over this type of self-testing, the results brought frustration over the negative impact it had on me. The adaptations themselves weren't the problem. It was the feelings of guilt that pushed me to go beyond reasonable limits, costing Kip and me a lot, both physically and mentally.

For the most part, I felt I was facing barriers almost too high for me to climb. I just couldn't figure out how to change things positively, acceptably. God remained faithful by my side, but He needed me to surrender my will, which I was obviously reluctant to do. I tried to go the direction I felt He was leading, yet somewhere along the way I seemed to get side-tracked, catching a glimpse of how I wanted things to turn out, subsequently letting go of His hand, stumbling miserably on my own.

I battled with all kinds of emotions inside. Loving the Lord Jesus with all of my heart, I passionately wanted others to witness God's provision for my life. My desire was genuine yet misguided, as I wanted them to see Christ through the ways I was managing this disability. It was very important to me to portray a Christian woman who could do anything through Christ, not a woman who remained focused on her problems while proclaiming to walk with Him.

I wanted to move on. I had always included the Lord in my efforts to seek out workable solutions to challenges in my life, yet during this particular divide in the road I seriously questioned the depth of my faith. No matter how hard I tried, I could not find concrete solutions to change what was happening. I was a Christian. I believed God could do the impossible, even when human diagnosis appeared grim. I had seen Him work miracles in others' lives. I considered that perhaps my belief for a miracle was weak. I prayed and prayed for my previous abilities to re-appear. So God would be glorified, and I would be "normal" again. Disappointment weighed heavily on my heart because they were not returning. I was losing focus of the reality of the situation, and it was resulting in a chaotic period of guilt and doubt.

I was afraid of being left out. I was also afraid for Kip. I didn't want him missing out on things because I had something "wrong" with me. We did enjoy private times of happiness and laughter as we spent time one on one with another person, or another couple. We didn't live in a cave of gloom. My reasoning and intellect were intact, and enjoying the company of just one or two lessened the struggles dramatically.

Group events were much more problematic, because of my newly imposed lack of understanding. The overwhelming madness of conversation and other visual and audible stimuli was unbearable. I quickly became unresponsive and extremely fatigued in these situations. A small nucleus of friends and loved ones who chose to grow with us were an enormous blessing. Kip and I really needed support, encouragement and understanding. I never once questioned my self-worth or value when in their presence. With them, I never had reason to. Their love carried both of us through the turbulent seas of unforeseen storms.

During the early phase of my diagnostic understanding, I tried to gently enlighten others about some of the challenges I was experiencing. My actions and reactions were often unusual, so I had been encouraged to let others know there would be definite changes in how I did things. This positive advice to educate brought encouragement initially; however, I quickly discovered that life's lessons don't always conform to the ideal.

I deeply desired to attend a special function. I prepared for it as best I could, trying to get adequate rest two days beforehand. I was somewhat apprehensive because I knew a lot of people would be present. Although I couldn't understand a lot of what was being said, I felt I managed the situation really well. There were many people engaged in varying conversations and while I couldn't join in, I was content with the blessing of being there, drinking it all in. Fatigue blanketed my body for three days following that event, yet I was so pleased I had attended.

Unfortunately, I had not been aware of a lack of expression on my face in group situations. This occurred because I couldn't process what was being said. A short time later, the blank look was painfully brought to my attention, along with my inability to converse, even though I had tried to explain my disability prior to attending. That painful awareness became a constant aching reminder of something precious I had lost, in more ways than one. My deepest desire had always been to radiate the joy of my relationship with Christ. I always believed a warm and genuine smile was the most visible and down-to-earth avenue to share that joy with others, even if words were not present. But I couldn't call it up. One of my favourite passages was Proverbs 15:30, *"A cheerful look brings joy to the heart, and good news gives health to the bones."*

From that moment of awareness, I worked so hard to have a cheerful look, but within minutes the effects of my brain injury erased any trace of it. I had to concentrate heavily on what was taking place and the scrambling of information would completely steal my energy reserve. The "vacancy" sign reappeared, and I felt foolish so many times as my heart echoed those painful words.

I had no marred physical, visible disability or handicap. Yet because of my unmarred physical appearance, erroneous beliefs surfaced which challenged the reality and seriousness of my brain injury. Misunderstandings were very painful, so I unwisely chose to ignore the new boundaries I had been advised to set, afraid of encountering additional losses. I repeatedly forced myself to step into situations that were unbearable for me. I often pushed myself to the point of almost passing out, ignoring the warning signs of blurred vision and nausea. I struggled unsuccessfully to mask the confusion and pain. I did not want to be set aside from partaking in life's events, nor did I want to be regarded as unkind, rude, uncaring, or—worst of all—selfish. Yet as hard as I tried, I was sometimes viewed as such and this broke my heart. I felt like a complete failure.

Fully knowing the consequences, I continued to venture unsuccessfully into areas of previous comfort and ease. I said yes to a lot of situations I could not cope with. Numerous times, however, I did not even realize the challenge involved until I was smack-dab in the middle of it. This was all so foreign to me. Everything was so unpredictable. I was un-expressive and I ran on empty for quite a long time. My body responded unfavourably to the impossible role I was demanding of it. Scrambling to find some type of consistency in my life, I tried to hide my struggles, deepening the ache inside of me while magnifying the futility of my efforts.

Because of the brain injury, I became "different" literally overnight. My limitations frustrated me because they were now a permanent part of who I was. I couldn't get rid of them and I couldn't hide them, despite my best efforts. I couldn't keep the disability to myself. It was re-shaping my life, and in effect would re-shape my relationships with others ... for a lifetime. The effects of my disability exposed themselves without reserve, as I had no control over how my brain responded to certain situations. In a busy mall setting, I would walk past someone I knew well without acknowledging them. When talking on the phone, I would unexpectedly hand it over to Kip without saying a word to the person on the other end. I just couldn't grasp what was being said. In the middle of conversation at a social event, I would suddenly leave with no explanation.

I really battled with feelings of guilt and shame. Of even greater concern to me was the odd ways my brain injury made me function. At times there was absolutely no graciousness in how I would react to certain situations. And, for the most part I did not recall what it was I had done until someone made me aware of it. Each and every time I attended a social function where several people were present I felt completely lost, appearing indifferent to conversations as my face mechanically produced a blank or perplexed look resulting from a lack of understanding of what was being said. I could hear voices talking, but the words and music resounded in my head, scrambling together like an orchestral warm-up before a concert. Nothing made sense. Sometimes barely making it to the car, I would inevitably be downhearted, embarrassed and in tears.

I struggled with tremendous guilt over my inability to participate in common everyday events with people I cherished, in the fashion most folks are used to. The fatigue from these outings would sap the energy from me for two or three days. I worried about Kip and the toll it was taking on him. Again, guilt flowed over me as I felt responsible for the events he was missing because of my disability. At one point, I questioned how long he would tolerate my inabilities.

I didn't realize during this tumultuous time what an enormous mistake I was making in my efforts to cover up the seriousness of my brain injury with others. I was so afraid of offending someone again. My stubborn resolve to try to carry on with life as usual when there was nothing usual to be found anymore was essentially backfiring on me, causing chaos, frustration and unrelenting confusion. It certainly didn't fix the problem. It likely intensified it.

I never anticipated how difficult it would be to accept this disability. If I remained in the quicksand of silence and insecurity, I knew I would be swallowed up by guilt, inner turmoil and ongoing frustration. Deep in my heart I desperately wanted to flourish beyond this stagnant place. I craved to grow past the limitations of this disability. I just didn't know how. Frankly, there were no concrete solutions or answers for the way I had to do things. Kip and I were still in the process of familiarizing ourselves with the brain injury itself, however it became evident that the process would never change. There would always be surprises and unexpected challenges. Adaptations would need constant evaluation. Medications would need to be continually monitored and adjusted for achieving the most effective results. What worked at one time would not necessarily continue to be effective down the road.

As I mulled over my options, certain truths slowly manifested themselves. I was tired of the turmoil and unwarranted feelings of guilt. The only way I could move past this barrier was to confront the question of why I struggled with such guilt. The answers were difficult, yet enlightening. I had self-imposed some unrealistic expectations, ignoring professional advice regarding the importance of setting and adhering to boundaries. Feelings of guilt would wash over me when I was harshly confronted by the effects of my willful disobedience to that advice. Proactive removal of those feelings of guilt was within reach. With God's help and guidance, I could ease the pressure I was putting upon myself.

Experiencing guilt in this form is justified when we willfully attempt to go beyond what God has enabled or empowered us to do. Our flippancy to replace God's boundaries with our own willful desire to go beyond them, particularly when searching for human acceptance, is sinful. We will become shallow if we seek to forego who we really are in order to meet someone else's expectations. Lost behind a mask of false pride, we are afraid to let others know about the weaknesses and imperfections that lurk in that vulnerable place. We fear judgment, criticism, ridicule or, even worse, rejection. It will cause us to fail time and time again. The only way out? To seek forgiveness, cleansing and renewal from the Father.

This form of guilt would also be warranted if the motive within our heart was to hurt, offend, or insult. But to remain within necessary boundaries for the sake of retaining personal health, with no intent to offend, is only indicative of a heart that recognizes the value of obedience to God's guidance. Through our obedience, God will provide positive alternatives to deepen healthy relationships.

But there was another side to the guilt I was experiencing. It was much, much more difficult to identify. When an illness or an accident brings change in any form, we often experience lack of understanding and/or lack of acceptance from others—even unknowingly. The need to place boundaries sometimes induces disappointment, and declining an invitation can be viewed as uncaring or selfish. When we do not take newly acquired limitations into consideration, customary expectations can become unrealistic. Since I was unable to meet those expectations, the heartache of regret manifested itself in the form of unwarranted guilt. The ability to meet them is simply just not there. It was here that I had to search deeply within my heart.

Harbouring feelings of guilt is wrong when expectations or circumstances are beyond our control, and our decision to remain within necessary boundaries is explained, yet not accepted. Declining to participate doesn't carry with it any intention to hurt if we genuinely try to give our very best. This kind of guilt is unwarranted and should be released to the Father with no string attached for retrieval.

Feelings of guilt and not measuring up were my biggest stumbling block. I needed to identify where my feelings of guilt and denial were coming from in order to find freedom. This part of the journey was going to be rough. The outcome would depend on my perseverance to prevail over unwarranted guilt. I needed God's guidance to do this, as only He could walk me through the foggy haze of justified guilt versus unwarranted guilt. Clearly understanding and recognizing each form of guilt would bring tremendous freedom and peace to my soul.

I continued to see doctors and specialists, becoming more confident in their genuine support and encouragement of my determination to find practical and successful ways of adapting to the challenges I was experiencing. Aware of the personal struggles I was having with guilt and frustration, advisors heavily stressed the importance of openly discussing my disability by explaining limitations, the need to pace myself, and the significance of monitoring each decision and circumstance. I would need to evaluate each situation before consenting to attend. They strongly emphasized that I needed to be absolutely okay within myself with the reasons behind necessary adaptations. For the sake of my health and Kip's, I needed to grasp the importance of incorporating self-evaluation into every decision I would make. Having the courage to make these types of choices would transpose apprehension into quiet confidence.

The constant support, guidance, firmness and forewarnings I received from these professionals slowly began to open the door of truth for me. I knew the consequences and I knew the pain of trying to fit back into a mould that was no longer suitable. Deep down in my heart, I really did know that the decisions I was making to avoid feelings of guilt could not continue. I was battling a war of acceptance. Trying to be the old me so I could acceptably fall in line with the rest of the world was essentially destroying the only me I had left.

I was slowly arriving at a place of allowing God to shed some light on why I was working so hard to push past my limitations. I would require constant guidance and counsel to figure out how to manage those feelings of guilt. There had been so much change since the accident that I knew

I could not sort out these feelings on my own. Gradually, a small seed began to sprout. Becoming proactive in how I dealt with my disability would entail much more than adaptations alone. Self-acceptance and self-assurance were the oars that would guide the effectiveness of my adaptations.

Opening my heart once again to the Lord, I sought His strength instead of my own. I sought His truth instead of frantically trying to fight the truth of my disability. Most importantly, I asked Him to help me grab hold of the enduring peace of His unconditional acceptance. God enabled me to recognize the STOP sign at the entrance of the dangerous pathway I had almost chosen to travel—a pathway I would have embarked on by ill choice, having let go of His hand.

I had been losing sight of my worthiness in God's eyes, seeking to find that worth in the world's eyes instead. I permitted Satan to whisper lies to me, telling me it was my responsibility to appear strong. He convinced me to depend on my inner strength alone. I became so focused on the lies he was telling me that I almost lost sight of my Father again. Satan continually whispered to me that I was letting others down, that I was weak, and that I must not reveal the complete effects of my disability because others may treat me differently and I would end up alone. He sought to use my human need for love and acceptance during a life-changing time to draw me away from the truths of Almighty God and His all-encompassing power and unconditional love.

What Satan was doing was symptomatic of a thief. He is an invisible thief who steals life, truly abundant life. A mislaid sense of self-worth burdened my heart as I listened to his lies. I did not want any part of him remaining within me. I sought total cleansing after finally recognizing the subtle power he had maliciously used to wreak havoc with my life following the accident.

As will happen countless times in any Christian's life, recognition of falling away called me to seek God's forgiveness. Again, I needed to be cleansed from doubt, fear, pride, and guilt. Yet again, I asked for His strength to renew my soul. His personal love flowed over me like a refreshing stream, revitalizing my weary and worn-out spirit. Isaiah 58:11 says, *"The LORD will guide you always; he will satisfy your needs in a sun-scorched land and will strengthen your frame. You will be like a well-watered garden, like a spring whose waters never fail."* My spiritual appetite was returning, and I found myself hungry for His vision.

Craving to know where God wanted to lead me, I searched the Scriptures. As with all sound counsel, I knew I needed to listen, then apply. Almighty God is by far the wisest and most compassionate Counsellor available. Access to Him is immediate and costs not even a penny. All God asks for is pure and complete trust in Him. Total faith. God's word is just that—His Word. He speaks to us through His Word. His wisdom is discerning and stalwart. Best of all, He instills life, truly abundant life.

2

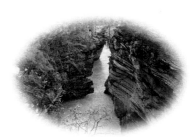

SURRENDERING GUILT

NEW BEGINNINGS WERE ON THE AGENDA AS I ONCE AGAIN PLACED MY LIFE into the Lord's care. I was eager for the teaching to begin. My disability had introduced me to such a foreign world that I kept gazing backward, hoping to avoid this unknown place in front of me.

Innocently enough, I had allowed Satan to cause incredible upheaval. I had been so focused on doing whatever was necessary to make feelings of guilt disappear that I did not recognize his interference. It didn't bother him in the least when I spoke to God. As long as I allowed frustration, guilt and doubt to fill my mind, it was okay with him. As long as I didn't call upon the name of Jesus to relinquish the turmoil these feelings were generating, Satan was satisfied with the job he was doing.

Surrendering once again to God was a direct threat to Satan, because he knew he could not succeed in his calculated efforts to continue the chaos in my life. James 2:19 confirms God's holiness and power: *"You believe that there is one God. Good! Even the demons believe that—and shudder."* I was ready to make Satan and his troops shudder! I opened my Bible and turned to 2 Timothy 1:7. As I soaked in each word, God reaffirmed to me the Holy Spirit's intervention when we allow Him access and when we ask Him to give us strength, courage and peace in who we are in Christ Jesus. This passage says, *"For God did not give us a spirit of timidity, but a spirit of power, of love and of self-discipline."* The Holy Spirit will empower us to live for God regardless of our circumstances, and will enable us to claim His power in all areas of our lives. He does not want us to be timid. He simply wants us to be obedient to His guidance.

God can only live and work in a subservient heart; He cannot live and work in a heart filled with self-focus and false pride. There is no room for God *and* self. True humility comes from recognizing the value and worth we have in God's eyes. It means having healthy self-esteem, understanding our self-worth because of the grace given to us through our Lord. Grace means finding favour in God's eyes. It cannot be earned—it is not even deserved. It is freely given simply because we are God's children. Our identity is wholly found in Christ Jesus. 1 Corinthians 15:10 says, *"But by the grace of God I am what I am, and his grace to me **was not without effect"*** (emphasis mine). God allows changes to take place in our lives for a specific reason.

The opposite of true humility is trying to be someone we cannot. Groping to find our worth in someone else's eyes initiates a completely false sense of pride. It also produces a sense of emptiness and continual searching. We will never be fully able to grasp the significance and value of our own lives in this way. Coming to terms with that, I searched for clarity of God's perspective on who I was so I would be able to serve His purpose the way He wanted. I would attain true humility when I fully recognized my worthiness in Christ alone. He had all of my days planned, including that moment of change on the highway in 2001. He knew before I was born that my life would take that turn. Psalm 139:2–3 says, *"You know when I sit and when I rise; you perceive my thoughts from afar. You discern my going out and my lying down; you are familiar with all my ways."* God was fully prepared to remain faithful each step of the way.

I could feel His love encompass me. Just as a blanket provides warmth and a sense of security, God wrapped Him arms of love around me. I praised Him for reminding me daily through His Word that I was not worthless, invaluable, useless or even less of a person because I had a disability that necessitated doing things differently. True humility does not mean putting ourselves down or allowing false guilt to invade our hearts. Those feelings of self-doubt will only yield destruction instead of freedom and confidence.

Scripture tells us that God gives *"a spirit of power, of love and of self-discipline"* (2 Timothy 1:7). God-given power enables me to roll up my sleeves and take on life with exuberance, limitations and all. Understanding God-ordained love allows me to recognize His perfect design from which He created me, giving me a much more secure sense of well-being, and facilitating me to share that same love with others. I require self-discipline to put on the brakes when I realize I am pushing myself too far because of unwarranted fears or guilt. I began to realize that God's power, along with His unfailing love, cannot illuminate from my life when the view I have of myself is distorted.

Looking to the Father first, and seeking His wisdom in making each and every decision, gave me a fresh and lively taste of the internal freedom that was available with those proactive decisions. Accountable to Him beyond all others, I became free to dispose of the guilt that still attempted to falsely whisper to me when I needed to retain certain boundaries. It is my responsibility to consciously rebuff any feelings of embarrassment in who I am, just as I am. Those feelings of embarrassment or shame are false. I am *His* child! It is wrong for me to submit to invalid guilt because my list of can and can't do's has changed due to my disability.

Hebrews 4:16 says, *"Let us then approach the throne of grace with **confidence**, so that we may receive mercy and find grace to help us in our time of need"* (emphasis mine). God was asking me to confidently approach His throne of grace every single time I sought His help. He doesn't want me approaching with my head hung low, my eyes lowered to the ground in shame. When asking forgiveness, yes, but when approaching Him for counsel, no. This was an awesome revelation for me.

Through much prayer and counsel, I am discovering that it is important for me to take proper care of myself for my own benefit, my husband's benefit, and the benefit of those I love so very much. Trying to go far beyond my newly acquired limitations weakens not only my body and mind, but my spirit as well. It also defies God's guidance and slowly opens the door just a crack for Satan to begin his attack once again. That's all he needs. Just a crack of self-doubt. Allowing him access of any kind significantly weakens my witness and overshadows my focus to possess that quiet strength which can only be evident through the self-assurance of who I am in Christ.

I have had to surrender my feelings of guilt, inadequacies, and wavering self-worth before the Lord many times, asking for His forgiveness. Forgiveness for the asking. Forgiveness given. Forgiveness to be received. Freedom in Christ is an indescribable, unconditional gift. It is available twenty-four hours a day, seven days a week. It begins with complete surrender to Christ. Precious time spent with my Lord strengthens me spiritually. Each time I surrender the sin of guilt and unworthiness, humbling myself before Him, I am cleansed, renewed, strengthened and more confident in being the woman He designed me to be.

Christ wants us to expect great things from Him. He demands reverence from us to recognize Him as Almighty God, Creator of all. We must never take His Omnipotence casually. Yet He is also our compassionate and loving Heavenly Father. He assures us of the confidence we can have in Him as Lord of our lives. 1 Peter 3:15 says, *"But in your hearts set apart Christ as Lord. Always be prepared to give an answer to everyone who asks you to give the reason for the hope that you have. But do this with gentleness and respect."*

This verse has a couple of key portions. We are told to set apart Christ as *Lord* in our hearts. We have no right as believers to place worry, fear, or guilt in that sacred place which is reserved for Him alone. When I uphold Him as Lord, I can have absolute confidence in Him, confidence in who I am in Him, and confidence in what He is going to do with my life. Confidence of this caliber increases through full trust in Him. It comes by believing in the certainty of His power. I must seek to do His will. I must willingly surrender my heart to His Holy Spirit for guidance. My mother wisely advises me to step back and take a good look at what He is doing right now in my life. Yes, He will be there tomorrow and the day after, but her counsel urges me to recognize His Presence within the hour, six hours or twenty-four hours right before me. When I heed that advice I become overwhelmed by God's display of love, and I am deeply encouraged by the Holy Spirit's recognizable activity.

Previously focused on the "underperformance" of my capabilities resulting from the brain injury, my confidence in myself, as well as Christ, had been severely shaken. In fact, I did not feel confident in anything for quite a while. I felt so lost, as though I had been plopped down in the centre of an enormous maze. Finding direction and purpose for my life seemed a world away. I battled endlessly with feelings of guilt as I fought ineffectively to regain my previous identity, hoping to end the frustration of perceived failure. Every time I tried to slip into my normal, everyday shoes, I ended up stumbling. They just didn't fit anymore.

God's Holy Word guided me to a renewed understanding that lack of (Christ-given) confidence does not have a place in healthy Christian living. I am His Child. He does not place conditions on the abundance of His love. He does not withhold it. Limitations, disabilities, arms, legs, eyes, ears, etc. are not qualifying factors for adoption into God's Kingdom. He created us and we are His children. His greatest desire is that we love Him in return, obediently following His commands. We are offered the incredible gift of eternal life with Him in His Heavenly Home, saved by grace alone through the blood of our Lord Jesus Christ when we accept Him as our Personal Saviour. Regardless of our appearance, capabilities or in-capabilities, we can journey through life with secure confidence in who we are through the blood Christ Jesus shed for us.

God's Word instructs that I must always be prepared to give an answer to everyone about what Christ is doing in my life and the hope for the future I have in Him. I was giving answers, but the wrong ones. Deciding to limit discussions about my disability after the first few discouraging attempts was a mistake. It was a decision based on fear of rejection along with unhealthy feelings of being different. My pride was also a factor. I didn't want the focus of conversation to be about me and the effects of this brain injury. I erroneously reasoned that if I didn't address it, it wouldn't become an issue.

I had hoped deep inside that no one would really notice the differences. I looked at myself in the mirror and saw no change physically except for the absence of the mischievous twinkle in my eyes. They had become dull and non-expressive, largely due to difficulties of trying to comprehend too much stimuli. I had hoped and prayed the internal differences that affected my external functions would mercifully disappear with time. Following the accident I was often asked, "How are you doing?" I would respond that I was doing fine and that there were only a few areas that needed time to heal. I became very uncomfortable when Kip would elaborate further, feeling like a stigma was then placed on my mental capacity. I was smart and didn't want to be viewed otherwise because people heard the words "brain injury."

These methods of handling situations backfired on me. I was intolerably aware of the problems that were bogging down my life, and I didn't want to stand around talking about them as well. I'm sure this caused confusion many times as I struggled to participate normally in situations that were impossible to function in. I attended but I didn't converse. I didn't converse because I *couldn't* converse. From the outside looking in, this may have created uncertainty as to why I did or didn't do certain things. New situations continued to arise and this disability was not an easy one to understand. Perhaps I wasn't comfortable discussing it because I still didn't know the extent of it. I was confused and didn't know how to handle the disability. Guilt was an eager companion when I didn't know how to address or respond to what was really happening inside of me. Instead of giving answers for the hope I had in Jesus, I was still pleading for answers from Him.

Taking those first steps to expose every part of myself to Jesus had been very difficult. It was a submissive decision in which I had to vulnerably admit that I was terribly lost, making mistake after mistake. As difficult as the exercise was, I counted on Him to meet me in that place of vulnerability, listening to and loving me through it. God lifted a tremendous burden from my shoulders as I sought His forgiveness then surrendered to His guidance. While seeking His truth, I was able to release much of the guilt I had been battling. It wasn't immediate. I felt the heaviness in my heart lighten, but I still had a long way to go. I was very aware that the decision to allow guilt access, or the decision to surrender it as soon as it threatened to infect me, would be a lifelong tug of war.

God's grace and patience with my stubbornness lessened the guilt trips each time I surrendered them. Coupling that with the guidance of other professionals and counsellors, I finally took the first step of my new journey as I focused on what God asked of me. I highly respected the counsel of my human advisors, but I could not succeed in sharing my faith through abundant living without my spiritual Counsellor, the Holy Spirit. Jesus alone made that transaction possible for me.

Finding confidence to openly discuss alternatives for various situations began allowing me to truly witness for Christ. I prayed frequently for confidence to override my innate desire to apologize for being unable to participate in something that was beyond my capabilities. I started to comprehend what it meant to willingly obey Christ. A stronger, healthier and happier lifestyle began to emerge as I came to recognize that doing less actually meant doing more. My adherence to new boundaries allowed me access to ground-breaking discoveries.

I found myself depending more and more on the Lord's strength, asking Him to shine through me. Constantly seeking His will, I no longer felt I had to prove I was in His care. Hebrews 12:2 says, *"Let us fix our eyes on Jesus, the author and perfecter of our faith."* I began to understand that when I have unwavering belief, there is no need to prove anything to anybody, including myself. There is only security and peace. The proof of surrender would reveal itself in the confidence and certainty of self.

I have always deeply desired for others to recognize Christ's Presence in my life. I've always wanted to radiate for Him. Genuine, continual interaction with Him confirmed that the best light He shines in is the light whose source is grounded in Him. To radiate for Christ, I must plug into the source of Life that gives life: God's Holy Word.

Deeper study unwrapped the blindfold of misinterpretation. True humility does not keep company with weakness or frailty of spirit, but instead stands firmly on the foundation of boldness and confidence found in a personal and intimate relationship with Christ Jesus. Boldness and confidence found through Christ Jesus is set apart from the worldly definition of those words. Aggressiveness, indifference, and self-gratification are not characteristics of spiritual boldness and confidence. Cradled in sensitivity, tenderness, certainty and self-worth, Christian boldness confidently radiates from within one's soul, defining an undeniable peace and contentment which only comes from the Holy Spirit.

A clearer sense of self evolves, paving the way to explore and set healthy boundaries. Most importantly, my boldness and confidence must reflect the personal relationship I have with Christ. Growth in discovering Christ-centered confidence can only result in gentleness, respect and humility as I move forward to share my life with others, exactly as it is. He has called me to share my life with others, adapting and making every effort possible to participate actively in their lives, where I can, whenever I can. As I progress, doors will begin to open, creating a deeper enjoyment of loved ones' lives because of my recognition to pace myself according to the signals transmitted by my brain. Time spent together will become far richer because "running on empty" will rarely be problematic.

Gently but confidently, I must try to provide answers that are sound and solid. Confidence will slowly replace guilt, even if the explanations I provide are not always understood or accepted. This new focus will encourage continued health to live my life with the refreshing peace of understanding and acceptance of who I am. I will *never* take for granted the unconditional faithfulness, understanding, compassion, encouragement, support and acceptance that flow from precious friends and loved ones who stand beside us, making the difficult task of adapting well worth the effort.

The love and faithfulness of these people have held Kip and me together when our life felt as though it was unravelling like a taut cord suddenly cut. The vast difference love and faithful support can make is emphasized in Ecclesiastes 4:12, *"Though one may be overpowered, two can defend themselves. A cord of three strands is not quickly broken."* Excellent Christian counsel alongside of the truths found in Scripture enabled me to understand that I am responsible for harbouring feelings of guilt that seemed to hold me captive. Feelings of guilt that seemed to drive me to do things I knew I shouldn't. Because I felt I had to. Those feelings of guilt were wrong and distracted me from doing what I knew was right and necessary to cope daily. Absorbed by fear and uncertainty of what others would think, I wrongly placed my focus on worldly self-worth.

Pushing myself past the point of my capabilities did not glorify God. Battling the belief that I was letting others down or that I was responsible for disappointing someone because I couldn't participate in something was creating a self-imposed false sense of guilt. Knowing the consequences and going against God's guidance triggered this type of guilt every time. However, my spiritual understanding was breaking down that barrier of lies. I began to understand that I was actually sinning against God because I was turning my back on His ultimate purpose for my life, seeking to define my own. The reason? I had tasted the bitter fruit of un-acceptance shortly after the accident, and it slammed me against a wall of confusion. To protect my heart I inwardly adopted the notion that I needed to push beyond my boundaries in order to be accepted, regardless of the damage these decisions were causing to the progress of my health.

I had acquired the belief that taking care of myself and pacing myself was selfish, when in fact *not* doing so produced many more problems than the actual disability. Wearing myself down to a broken heap, trying to prove to myself and others that I was capable of something I was not, did not honour God. Trying to do the impossible was preventing me from participating in healthy activities. My energy reserve quickly depleted as I continually put myself in situations that overloaded me to the point of extreme exhaustion and tears. Stress greatly added to the equation.

As I unwrapped my confusion before God, He gently washed my eyes with the salve of truth. Self-examination of the source of guilt is healthy and necessary. Guilt which arises from deliberate wrongdoing has its rightful place within the life of a Christian. But guilt which slinks in under false pretense and is permitted to slip onto the throne of my heart, even temporarily, is also wrong. And it is sinful.

Going to God's Word or communing with the Lord gives clearer insight to the validity and source of the guilt. A genuinely repentant heart is necessary in both cases for cleansing and renewal. Only then can I go before God Almighty with confidence, asking Him to deal with Satan's intrusion into my life. Seeking forgiveness, I can be bold in my request to prevail against it another time. Regardless of the form of guilt, God's promise stands. Sincere repentance of sin, either intentional or unintentional, frees me to move forward, clean and whole in the gift of life God has placed before me. From there, the responsibility remains in my court to let others know I would never intentionally hurt them, hopeful that understanding will replace misunderstanding.

I must not revert to shrinking away from facing the truths of my limitations head-on (no pun intended). Seeking to be proactive, my responsibility is to accept the changes in my life. I need to work with the changes, not fight against them. I must be confident when explaining the limits of my disability to others, and I must be bold in adhering to those limits without feeling guilt-ridden, uncomfortable or ashamed. My answers must be gentle and loving, yet firmly and confidently grounded. A lot of factors will determine each decision, and those factors will change constantly for a lifetime. My responsibility for accountability ends there. That advice seemed harsh, yet it was crucial. I cannot and must not assume responsibility for another person's thoughts, actions or responses. Acceptance of my decision lies in the hands of the other person. Where there is love, acceptance and complete trust, there is no need to question.

Choosing to make decisions with a spirit of determination blanketed by wisdom has allowed me to make sound choices while still challenging myself to grow and persevere. Hebrews 10:35–39 says,

So do not throw away your confidence; it will be richly rewarded. You need to persevere so that when you have done the will of God, you will receive what He has promised. For in just a very little

while, "He who is coming will come and will not delay. But my righteous one will live by faith. And if he shrinks back, I will not be pleased with him." But, we are not of those who shrink back and are destroyed, but of those who believe and are saved.

What an incredibly exciting passage! Paul emphasizes the divine significance of believing in what God can and will do! I can possess secure confidence in who I am in Jesus! Not in who I am alone, just as Kathie. How hollow that would be! God commands that I live by faith, not bound by shackles of endless limitations. Paul points out that this healthy and personal relationship with God will never allow for spiritual destruction. He does not want me to shrink back, adulterated by fear, shame, helplessness and unwarranted guilt. Trusting His Word and His promises with all my heart instills security and confidence in who I am as a child of God. Disability and all.

Allowing myself to question why I was experiencing such tremendous guilt after the onset of this disability helped clear the debris which had been constantly tripping me up. God was very patient with me as I worked hard to do the things He needed me to do in order to attain the freedom He promised. I still had a lot to learn, but another stepping stone toward a brighter future had provided me significant stability. Optimism was on the horizon.

3

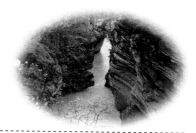

LETTING GO

I HAD BEGUN TO ACKNOWLEDGE THE CERTAINTY OF THE CHANGES that were now forming a new me, a term some specialists used. I found that term so difficult to relate to. I didn't want to be a new me, because I knew God had uniquely created *me* from the beginning. The only time I was comfortable becoming new was when I became a new creation in Him, accepting Him as Lord of my life. This is described in 2 Corinthians 5:17, *"Therefore, if anyone is in Christ, he is a new creation; the old has gone, the new has come!"* Becoming a new me in this spiritual sense was exciting because I willingly chose to leave behind anything that would hinder my walk with Christ. I publicly accepted Him as Lord of my life, renouncing the things which might lead me into the temptation of sin again. In making this decision, I became a new creation, forgiven and cleansed to start fresh with Christ's will as my sole focus.

The thought of having to identify with a new me, not by choice this time but by harsh circumstance, was definitely unsettling. Within my personal sense of reasoning, there were no physical signs that the old me had disappeared. I looked the very same. Yet I was so afraid of how others would view me. My disability was essentially indiscernible, with nothing to visually identify it. How then could anyone, including myself, accept a new me?

God had so much patience with me. Encouragement from professionals to openly grieve the loss of who I once was did prove to be extremely valuable in the healing process. I candidly admitted that "grieving the loss of who I was" sounded extremely strange to me. I was still alive, so what do I grieve for? What do I grieve about? As a Christian, was it wrong to grieve over my losses when I knew God had allowed the changes to take place? What does the word grief itself really mean? I hadn't been aware that I was already going through various stages of grieving. Tears, frustration, sorrow, guilt and anger disclosed a story laced with grief. Anguished, I had frantically tried to put back together the pieces that had erupted my identifiable life of forty-one years. I had previously known who I was, where I was going and what my life was about (or at least I thought I did). Within seconds, all of that certainty changed. Permanently.

I found myself looking in the mirror, staring at my familiar face, yet asking myself so many questions about who I was. It was difficult, very difficult to visually see the same person, exactly the same, looking back at me, tears streaming down her face. I yearned for answers as to why I couldn't move past these new roadblocks of limitations and enormous changes in my life. My incessant attempts to fall back into the familiar pattern of my life, along with feelings of guilt and frustration, bore clear medical evidence of the grief I was experiencing. After in-depth testing and counselling, several professionals concluded that I was not clinically depressed. I was, however, grieving the loss of who I had been prior to the accident. I did not recognize the process I was going through, but over time, counselling and discussions with professionals clarified what it meant to grieve the loss of who I was. I was encouraged to allow myself to grieve, as it was extremely beneficial for moving forward with my disability.

I had been trying to cover up my fears, my tears, my frustrations and my feelings of helplessness. Not always successfully in public, and seldom successfully at home. I was already experiencing grief, but had interpreted it as weakness, failure and a lack of faith because my clouded understanding of grief only pertained to someone physically passing away. The fog of misunderstanding began to lift as I became enlightened to the truth that grief slips into life in a variety of ways. Feelings of sorrow, heartache, and anguish all portray the very essence of grieving. Once I identified this reality, I knew I could only continue through this process holding tightly to my Lord's reassuring hand. My disability was no longer a masked stranger, but the temptation to keep looking back played havoc with my emotions. Many times I believed I had succeeded in dealing with acceptance. And, there were times when I truly had. But the whispers of what used to be continued to grate my resolve, and I'd find myself unsettled once again.

This emotional rollercoaster was a ride I'd never experienced before. My continual and optimistic outlook eliminated the possibility of clinical depression, for which I was tested three times by various professionals, including psychologists, psychiatrists, and neuropsychologists. Besides that medical confirmation, I knew I wasn't suffering from depression. I looked forward to each day, and despite all the rough spots, my determination to move forward remained constant.

It was time to clarify and address the grieving symptoms. Developing an understanding of this process was a critical step toward recovery. I began to realize that the continual error of looking back was causing me to trip and stumble in my efforts to move forward. I needed to let go. I needed to release my clutch on the false hope of restoration that was weighing me down. I needed to surrender my grief completely to God, asking Him to remould me as He wished, counting on Him to keep alive the qualities of my spirit and character that He most wanted for His purpose.

Letting go, surrendering all to God, was a very vulnerable place to enter. Giving it all to Him. I felt as an unformed ball of clay waiting to be remoulded into something new. I needed to rely on Him to help me confront the temptation to revisit memories of what I used to do, how well I used to do it, and the regrets of what I could no longer do. It was important to surrender comparisons of my prior capabilities with my newly induced limitations.

I didn't want to remain trapped in the vault of grief. Grieving was important and definitely had its place. Working through it strengthened me. I wanted and needed to be set free to discover new horizons. I knew I would continue to trip and stumble if I persisted in looking backward, wishing for something I could not have. That decision would allow the grief to remain and would continue to prevent me from becoming the woman God wanted and intended for me to be.

Following the accident, feelings of helplessness washed over me more times than I care to remember. Highs and lows of emotions seldom seemed to ease up. Even though I was enlightened as to why the tears and heartaches were taking place, the grieving process would take time. It was a process. Complete surrender to the Lord didn't occur overnight. It couldn't. Unidentified circumstances kept springing up before me, almost on a daily basis. I awoke every morning with anticipation for the new day, asking the Lord to be with me and to help me work through whatever came my way. He never left my side; however, He did not always intervene when situations or circumstances overwhelmed me. I guess there were certain things He knew I needed to experience. If He always came to my aid, I would not grow stronger nor would I be refined.

I have experienced the dark valley of being completely broken before God. It is a place of utter helplessness. One situation in particular literally brought me to the floor in a flood of tears. I ached inside crying out to God, wanting to know how I could have failed so badly in this area. An unrelenting battle was continuing to wage war as I tried so hard to live life as "normally" as I could. Yet the constant, unmasked reality of my disability's inadequacies was always raising its ugly head.

During this very low point in my life, Almighty God tenderly confirmed that He truly does hear our prayers and our moaning out to Him. In these critical moments, I personally experienced Him reaching down, holding out His hand to me. Not visibly or literally, but beyond a shadow of a doubt I was blanketed with His Holy Presence. He was there, right there with me. In my heart I heard Him say, "Take my hand, Kathie. Let's face this together. I'm right here with you."

Psalm 18:16 affirms the very essence of my experience: *"He reached down from on high and took hold of me; He drew me out of deep waters."* 2 Corinthians 4:7–9 describes God's powerful freedom beautifully, *"But we have this treasure in jars of clay to show that this all-surpassing power is from God and not from us. We are hard pressed on every side, but not crushed; perplexed, but not in despair; persecuted, but not abandoned; struck down, but not destroyed."* As God's children, we lay claim to the victory of freedom we have in Christ, allowing us to surrender our grieving. Through that victory we are free to celebrate the life God chooses to bless us with!

I immediately went downstairs and shared with my husband what had transpired. Then we prayed. We prayed and prayed, both releasing rivers of tears, holding each other, allowing God's comforting blanket of love to fill and restore our hearts so we could face the silent pain of this experience head-on with His guidance, strength and courage. It was a pivotal moment and a positive opportunity to move forward with a renewed spirit.

I believe God is very wise in His timely guidance. Someone brought to my attention at one point a situation where I had expressed anger along with unbridled sobbing over the fact that I had this life-altering disability while the individual responsible walked away virtually unscathed. The tears I readily released as I acknowledged my agonizing sorrow for a situation I had not caused were probably also a gift from God. A situation which crudely introduced a permanent disability into my life at the age of forty-one.

It was another step in letting go which God had granted at a specific time. This release was followed by a healthy understanding instead of angry hostility. Had I harboured that anger, dark feelings of bitterness would have taken root, and grown. I specifically had to bow before the Lord, seeking His power to completely remove any feelings of unforgiveness or resentment which I may have subconsciously harboured against this individual. I also asked Him to protect my heart from future resentment which may lurk around in my subconscious mind.

God powerfully reminds us of our responsibility to forgive, at all times. There is no more vivid example of this command to forgive than was illustrated at the cross. As He hung on the cross, cruelly wounded and taunted, our Lord Jesus Christ cried out to God Almighty, *"Father, forgive them, for they do not know what they are doing"* (Luke 23:34). People sneered at Him, scoffing at His pain. They laughed, mocking His claim to be the Messiah, God in the flesh. Yet, as commanded by His Father, Jesus asked forgiveness, for the entire world's sin.

Stephen witnessed boldly about Christ and His Oneness with God. This angered those who had condemned Christ for proclaiming to be God's Son. Because of their anger and their false sense of holiness, these men grabbed hold of Stephen and dragged him out of the city. They began to stone him for blaspheming against God. Stephen, even in his last moments before death, was an obedient servant, displaying a courage which verified his love and conviction in Who Christ is. Acts 7:59–60 recounts Stephen's last moments and words: *"While they were stoning him, Stephen prayed, 'Lord Jesus, receive my spirit.' Then he fell on his knees and cried out, 'Lord, do not hold this sin against them.' When he had said this, he fell asleep…"*

God calls me to forgive, regardless of situation or circumstance. He does not promise that everything will turn out fine because we have forgiven, but He does promise freedom from the bondage of an unforgiving heart. As I read the above passages, all I could think was, "How can I not forgive someone?" My disability is real and it has changed my life drastically. I will have struggles and challenges along the way. But I refuse to carry the excess baggage of an angry, unforgiving heart. When I forgive and when I seek forgiveness, immense freedom floods over my soul, bringing about a peace that is truly beyond all understanding. Words simply cannot explain the divine freedom that takes place. It is my full responsibility to genuinely forgive, whether it is accepted, rejected or met with indifference, regardless of the wrong which was done. Only God has the authority to judge another person.

Matthew 6:14–15 clarifies God's command to forgive: *"For if you forgive men when they sin against you, your heavenly Father will also forgive you. But if you do not forgive men their sins, your Father will not forgive your sins."* Ouch! That's a very powerful and humbling statement. I know I am a sinner who lets God down time and time again. Sometimes I am not even aware of my sin or perhaps the pain it has caused someone else. I need to bow before Almighty God, seeking His forgiveness for any sin I've committed which has let Him down. I also need to set free whomever I have felt has sinned against me, forgiving them while surrendering the pain to my compassionate Heavenly Father. This is not always easy to do. In fact, this is one of the most difficult steps of obedience to take. To be forgiven, I must forgive. It's that straightforward in God's eyes.

I have direct access to God, and may come before Him at any time. Jesus paid for that freedom through His death on the cross. Understanding my need for forgiveness as well as my need to forgive establishes feelings of profound gratitude and compassion. Forgiveness becomes a wrecking ball, as it completely destroys unseen walls built by resentment and anger. The freedom that results provides closeness with God that can only come from being purified by Him.

Being cleansed and renewed does not give me the right to pass judgment on anyone else. It does not place me a in a cleaner, spotless place where I can look down on others. Experiencing freedom from the bondage of sin must not remain self-contained. God forgives my sins, and I am free. It doesn't end there. Whatever I have done or said or thought has been forgiven by my Father when I genuinely sought His forgiveness. I am commanded to do no less for another, thus being called to sincerely forgive, surrendering any root of bitterness to the Lord. Doing so unlocks the chains Satan tries to bind around my soul. I can only be cleansed if my heart does not harbour resentment toward another.

Sure enough, we all have had times when we have been innocently, accidentally, or intentionally hurt by others, physically and/or emotionally. If we don't release the pain and anger to God our Father, we remain as prisoners of bitterness and our lives will never experience the joy and freedom that comes from true forgiveness. I don't want to stay there, in the cesspool of anger. Life would be empty and void of true joy, and I would be as guilty as the one I am continuing to accuse. Letting go of the hurt and pain through forgiveness obeys God's command. Certain situations or circumstances may not ever change, but God keeps

His promise of instilling a deep and lasting joy that can only come from a heart free of bitterness and anger.

I had the opportunity to meet the individual who hit my van. I was apprehensive at first. I felt sure I was not holding any bitterness against him. I had had my open release that one particular time. However, I was still concerned. I wondered that morning if seeing him, or hearing what he might say, might trigger some subconscious, unknown feelings of anger I thought I had surrendered. I can only say that during our short meeting, God's Holy Spirit was abundantly present and Satan's whispers of doubt were replaced by a tremendous and powerful sense of peace. I walked out of the room entirely free to move into the future. It was an amazing revelation of God's faithfulness in keeping His promises.

We need to remain attentive to God's leading. He will help us recognize His timing, and He encourages us to step out in faith holding fast to His hand. He doesn't want us to pull back fearfully, nor rush ahead of His guidance. We need to let go of our grip on the past in order to move forward with our hand placed in His. He requires trust. Complete trust! 2 Corinthians 4:16–18 encourages us to focus on the victory we have in Christ:

> *Therefore we do not lose heart. Though outwardly we are wasting away, yet inwardly we are being renewed day by day. For our light and momentary troubles are achieving for us an eternal glory that far outweighs them all. So we fix our eyes not on what is seen, but on what is unseen. For what is seen is temporary, but what is unseen is eternal.*

How intimate is our Lord! It is His Word that tells us to fix our eyes on things unseen, which are eternal, rather than placing our focus on things which we can only humanly see with limited understanding. He counsels us that what is seen is temporary. He also tells us that what has been is temporary.

Knowing this speaks of our spiritual relationship with Him, of our promise for eternal life with Him in Heaven. His Word is comforting, but it is also vibrant and alive, and declares the hope and power which flows down from God Almighty. There are many, many challenges facing those with disabilities, both visible and invisible. God calls us to fix our eyes on Him. He beckons us to let go, trading the limitations of our mortal bodies for the victory we can claim in Him, which will last forever. What is seen is temporary and has the potential to change at any given time. Yet our souls are eternal—who we are is eternal. Our God is such a personal God, and He has given all of us a spirit that cannot be touched by any disability or any circumstance!

He has promised to always walk through the valley of grief with His children. I believe what is discovered and released in the depths of that valley refines and purifies us. Surrendering everything to Jesus, completely letting go, withholding nothing, we become thoroughly cleansed deep down inside. As spotless as an untouched canvas, willing and ready to be used by God. Take a moment to really think about that! To be used by God Almighty! He is the artist, and He is the One Who chooses to give our lives worth and beauty regardless of the circumstances we find ourselves in. We need only to follow His guidance, draw on His strength, and recognize our value and worth in His eyes.

4

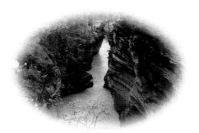

CONQUERING DOUBT

DOUBT DIVERTS FEELINGS OF CERTAINTY, TRUST, BELIEF AND CONFIDENCE from the peaceful waters of a focused faith into a dark whirlpool of turmoil and confusion. Darkness begins to hover over us, making our focus dim, foggy, harder to see. Even when we have surrendered, accepted, and decided resolutely to move forward, the slightest seed of doubt can churn the still waters.

Doubt robs our peace and occurs when we rely on our own human capabilities or reasoning. James 1:5–6 says, *"If any of you lacks wisdom, he should ask God, who gives generously to all without finding fault, and it will be given to him. But when he asks, he **must believe** and **not doubt**, because he who doubts is like a wave of the sea, blown and tossed by the wind"* (emphasis mine). Living in the chaos of doubt, tossed by the wind and waves, wanes our confidence in God. Not completely trusting Him is suggestive of relying on myself and what I envision the results to be. It does not keep my hand placed in the Father's, but instead indicates that I am letting go ever so slightly, uncertain He truly can change things.

One day, I was telling my mother about a situation I was really struggling with. I shared with her how passionately Kip and I had been praying about it. It was a serious matter and I asked her how we would recognize God's answer. In her wisdom she simply said, "Because you asked Him with a sincere heart." No secret potion. No magic wand. No crystal ball. Just a genuine request for understanding.

Achieving true faith and trust in our personal, loving God transpires when we believe without doubt that He hears our voices and sincere hearts. His promise stands true that He hears our genuine prayers. Psalm 66:16–20 declares,

> *Come and listen, all you who fear God; let me tell you what he has done for me. I cried out to him with my mouth; his praise was on my tongue. If I had cherished sin in my heart, the Lord would not have listened; but God has surely listened and heard my voice in prayer. Praise be to God, who has not rejected my prayer or withheld his love from me!*

When our hearts are genuinely seeking Him, He will hear our prayers.

Seeking His Word and His wisdom connects me directly with my Lord. Sometimes I have wondered if Satan can whisper things to me, confusing me, making me question if an answer is from God or not. But my mother taught me that when we pray with a sincere heart to God, Satan may try to intervene; however, his efforts will be in vain when we place our focus on Christ, completely trusting Him. God's Holy Word validates that lesson. James 4:7–8 says, *"Submit yourselves, then, to God. Resist the devil, and he will flee from you. Come near to God and He will come near to you…"*

His answers may not always come right away, may not always be on our schedule, may not always be what we want to hear, but He will answer a sincere believer's heart who desires His will, not their own. 1 John 5:14–15 says, *"This is the confidence we have in approaching God;*

that if we ask anything according to His will, He hears us. And, if we know that He hears us—whatever we ask—we know that we have what we asked of Him."

Growing stronger spiritually, I have discovered true delight in the arrival of each day and the promises it holds, even though I have no idea what lies ahead. I hold onto the promise that He will guide me through each day. I think about all the wonderful things to be accomplished. When doubts do come, and they always will, I once again go to the Lord in prayer and read His Word.

Galatians 6:4–5 emphasizes, *"Each one should test his own actions. Then he can take pride in himself, without comparing himself to somebody else, for each one should carry his own load."* This passage seems to cut to the very core of the biggest challenges I've experienced. This very verse could easily summarize the initial reason for my writing this book. Comparison, whether it is to someone I used to be, or to others' capabilities, renders a most unsatisfactory and dismal future. It redirects my focus, allowing the potential for doubt to slyly sneak in. Instead, I am instructed to test my own actions. I am instructed not to compare! No matter what situation or circumstance I encounter. Of importance is what I do with the situation before me. It means touching base with the Lord for guidance first, then carrying myself to do the task to which I am called. Not someone else, me! What I needed to understand and accept is that the decision I make is the best decision for who I am.

Doubt usually takes the form of questioning myself, comparing my present capabilities to pre-accident state. God is not interested in these comparisons. They evolve solely within the human mind. They can only exist if I feed them. I must choose to shake them off their unstable footings if I am to grow in character. Realigning my focus is crucial to quickly dissolving feelings of doubt. I must release these comparisons and concentrate on the truth that God can use me regardless of my limitations. This helps strengthen my confidence in Christ, and myself. His love can radiate through my life to others, and confidence in who I am encourages others to accept me as I am because I display more certainty, more sureness in my interaction with them.

Love is not impaired by limitations or a disability. Christ truly conquers doubt and increases feeling of self-worth when we earnestly seek His will. Romans 8:26–27 says,

In the same way, the Spirit helps us in our weakness. We do not know what we ought to pray for, but the Spirit himself intercedes for us with groans that words cannot express. And he who searches our hearts knows the mind of the Spirit, because the Spirit intercedes for the saints in accordance with God's will.

Eliminating doubt requires daily assessment of my focus. Although I would love to never encounter feelings of doubt again, I am very aware of my humanness, and so is Satan. He lingers around eagerly ready to seize his prey. Close communion with Almighty God readjusts my spiritual armour, protecting my spirit from Satan's lies. I grow each time I surrender those doubts to the Lord, accepting His confirmation of my worthiness. Then, I must close that door.

Doubt cannot linger if it is not fed. We must go beyond seeking. We must follow through to being proactive. Remaining trapped in the mud of questions and doubt, asking the same questions over and over without actively pursuing and accepting answers, will swallow us up. We will sink into an emotional place of unhealthy bitterness. I continue to ask God for His help and strength so I can skip through the muddiness of doubt instead of becoming entrapped in it.

5

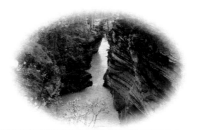

Overcoming Loneliness

Loneliness whispered quietly in my heart at times, especially once I had to accept that I could no longer work at the shop, nor participate in certain social activities. The flurry of interaction which had been present on a daily basis diminished rapidly. Being in the hub of activity was no longer possible and I missed it a great deal, particularly in the first three years following the accident.

It's crucial for me to be aware of an important event well ahead of time. I must consider many factors, such as the time of the event, physical surroundings and possible medication adaptations. Extreme sensitivity to noise and busyness greatly limits my interaction with others within any activity which is…active. Even attending church requires adaptations such as slipping in after the service starts and leaving just prior to the close of the service. Words are jumbled as folks greet each other and I cannot sort out multiple conversations, let alone become involved in any. I experience this in all group activities, which severely limits my involvement.

I have always been a curious gal. I enjoy knowing how and why things work the way they do. I love to research and investigate. I began searching for tangible solutions from books and literature written about mild traumatic brain injuries. These were extremely helpful aides which introduced me to positive methods of learning how to further adapt to the challenges I was facing and would continue to face. Practical suggestions lit the fire of personal exploration. I write everything down on sticky notes, whiteboards, and computer calendars to combat memory challenges. To provide uniformity, recurring appointments are scheduled for the same day of the week, at the same time. Games such as Scrabble Flash and Yahtzee stimulate and challenge my brain. Word search books force me to concentrate as I seek out singular words in a maze of jumbled letters.

Research also suggested that seventy to ninety percent of the people involved in my life prior to the brain injury may draw away from the relationship they had with me, or relationships would change depending on others' willingness to adapt with me. This is largely due to lack of understanding of the disability. Personally, I believe it is also a reaction to uncertainty, not really knowing what to make of my disability because it is not a visible handicap. This type of withdrawal is not intentional, it is just part of our human nature. According to one head trauma specialist, feelings of loneliness are extremely common among people who suffer from the effects of a brain injury. The changes definitely cause uncertainty for everyone involved. Many marriages suffer immensely. Many do not survive.

God knew I was a social butterfly. He knows I still am. He's moulded that personality into who I am. I pondered over how I was going to overcome these times of loneliness. My heart pleaded with my emotions, begging me to participate in events as they arose. I felt as though I was caught in the middle of a tug of war, my heart and emotions craving to join the fun, my brain and disability stating bluntly that I could not.

Once again, I went to my Creator asking for guidance. I laid all my cards on the table, exposing my dilemma. Proverbs 18:24 spoke to my heart. It says, *"A man of many companions may come to ruin, but there is a friend who sticks closer than a brother."* I took a long time reviewing this verse, asking God for wisdom in understanding its message. Authentic fellowship was His reply. Genuine, precious, intimate fellowship. This verse encouraged me to explore my treasure chest of friendships.

This exercise reminded me of the friends and family members who have remained bonded to Kip and me throughout the turmoil of changes. I envision it this way: as we go through troubled waters with the seas raging all around us, there are those who will stand on the shore and cheer us on. The waters get higher and the storm fiercer. The cheers encourage us to keep fighting the tumultuous sea, but the voices gradually fade as the storm rages on. We feel alone, almost overwhelmed by the torrents of challenges threatening to destroy us. We sense we are drowning in seas of uncertainty, sorrow, bewilderment, confusion and frustration. We can no longer see nor hear the ones who remained safe on the shore of familiarity.

But wait. One hand, then two, three, four... reaching out for us to grab onto, arms pulling us up to the top again, words of loyalty and faithfulness flowing from the mouths of those who have chosen to ride the sea of turmoil right alongside of us. Brothers and sisters who are committed to being there when they are needed the most. Jumping into our storm of life as if it were theirs. No questions, no judgments, no conditions. Only simple, wonderful and unconditional love that says, "I'm here for you, no matter what life brings your way." Recognizing and appreciating the priceless treasure we have with those closest in our lives speaks again of God's faithfulness and eases the heartache that loneliness brings. Gratitude for what I do have instead of hungering for what is missing has helped me let go of the *need* to be around others.

Unconditional love will never wander. Spending time together, one on one with another person or with one couple is intimate and extremely rewarding. Friends have shared with us how refreshing it is to be able to enjoy a special type of fellowship in this way, instead of the surface talk they experience at times in large gatherings. This is the unmatched quality of friendship that says, "I'm really glad you are here and I enjoy the depth of fellowship we share."

The process of being open to learning initiates valuable lessons. At various points in this journey forward, I often discover one of my original gifts still intact. As the requirement for a certain gift arises, often spontaneously, I marvel at the wonderful truth that God really is faithful. I am slowly discovering how He has protected many of my original gifts. He has also preserved my character and personality. Daily living still presents challenges I've never encountered before, but the core of who I am deep inside still remains.

Trustworthiness fits into that category. I can be trusted. I have always been trustworthy, and this quality has been the glue cementing deep, deep friendships. Unhurried time spent with someone allows trust to develop. Trust—deep, genuine trust—flows from one heart to another. Because my life is quieter and slower paced now, I am in a unique position to share precious time with others in a way that the world forfeits because of busyness, stress and worry. Matthew 18:20 says, *"For where two or three come together in my name, there am I with them."* Focusing on another's need in a serene, unrushed, quiet place is not commonplace in today's society. "Time" doesn't allow for such a luxury. Yet such a place of quietness promotes self-renewal.

Unforeseen blessings have also showered down on us through the gift of newly acquired friendships. These human treasures have come into our lives in effect because of my disability. They are aware of my disability, although they may not completely understand it. Some had not known me prior to the accident, therefore they have nothing in the past to compare me to. My life as it is now is the only way they have ever known me. This provides so much freedom for me to just be me. Not long ago, a fairly new and cherished friend of mine expressed her admiration of how much I am able to do, how far I've come since she has known me. Her sincere and encouraging words gave me a beautiful gift that day, the reassurance of how God is blessing my life.

Long-term friendships which have endured the challenges and joys along with us are more precious than jewels. Those friends' willingness to work through the changes with us touches our hearts beyond words. We hold on tight to the priceless gifts of love from the ones who are willing to just simply accept. They know my limitations and respect them.

Visits may be somewhat shorter, but the time of sharing together is very fulfilling. Now, several years after the accident, we are attempting to entertain a bit more, letting understanding and knowledge guide our times of fellowship. Friends recognize the oncoming fatigue. I do not need to explain why I slip away when I am overloaded. Fellowship continues with Kip, and I may or may not return depending on how quickly I recharge. The continual visits, coupled with love and acceptance, warm our home and our hearts, encouraging us to press on with solutions that once again enable us to entertain, in unique ways.

This is a process, and loneliness still knocks at my heart's door. Family gatherings and holidays are joyous events and usually involve large groups of people with festive music and lots of activity. What fun to share the joyful times that bring sheer delight to everyone involved! After all, these times cry out for celebration! However, these events can silently raise my loneliness meter a notch or two. My heart wishes I didn't have to quietly slip away from the celebrations shared with loved ones, nevertheless I would never wish to dampen or alter events. My decision needs to be carefully thought through before accepting an invitation to these.

I am appreciating the necessity of letting certain folks know (such as the hosts) that I may have to leave early, and why. In most cases there is warm understanding. Through prayer and acceptance, I am learning to tuck the joy I've encountered into my heart as I slip away to a more restful place, endeavoring to be content with what I have been able to share in. I am also learning to consciously leave the destructive shadow of discontentment outside my door. I continue to pray for acceptance of the methods I must use to cope during an event, whether it is slipping away quietly, being present for only a short period of time, or graciously declining an invitation altogether as a result of various circumstances.

I am still searching for alternatives. I always will be. God is teaching me to adapt in really neat ways. I can attend weddings, but wedding receptions are more unpredictable. I can go to church, but I need to monitor my attendance according to the activities involved each time. Having guests over primarily in the mornings, for breakfast or brunch, seems to be working very well, as my medication is most effective at that time and I feel my best after a good night's sleep. As events arise I make every effort to participate, but exceptions need to accepted as just that—exceptions. There will always be the possibility that I will not be able to prepare for, or attend, spontaneous activities.

Discoveries of successes versus the disappointment of failure have evolved only through trial and error. The only way to learn what I can and cannot accomplish is by attempting to do something, be somewhere or participate in an event only to discover that I pay heavily for that particular decision for several days afterward. The answer then has become very clear. But it is this process that is helping me understand what is possible and what is not. I do need to be certain I have tried all possible methods before turning down an opportunity for fellowship. I'm not interested in nursing the potential for loneliness as a self-inflicted wound.

Traditionally, Christmas is a time of celebration. Planned activities swirl around on calendars, announcing that busy is best. Yet, Christmas can be an extremely challenging and lonely time of year for people with disabilities. I have only truly recognized this since acquiring my own disability.

As Christmas approached the year after my accident, I found myself secretly wishing it was all over. I didn't want my precious husband or family to know of my insecurity. I was extremely concerned about how I was going to manage all the interaction. I didn't want to put a damper on festivities by revealing my perceived weaknesses and limitations. Limitations that would affect time spent with them. Realistically, I couldn't understand what was being said in large gatherings and I dreaded the difficulty of going shopping even though my heart craved to find special items. I was fearful of the fellowship that revolved around us as celebrations began, knowing I couldn't understand what was going on, knowing I couldn't participate comprehensibly. I desired to interact with loved ones but was missing out on so much of the joy.

Loneliness and frustration washed over me. I was apprehensive as to how I could cope with so much activity. I was profoundly aware that if we didn't participate, there would be a high possibility of experiencing a sense of isolation. I just couldn't do that to my husband at that special time of year we both loved so very much. We had been engaged Christmas Eve, 1978, and Christmas has always held very special memories. Kip's constant love wrapped around me endlessly during the struggles of that first Christmas season. He always considered the price I would pay if I proceeded beyond my capabilities. He also didn't want to attend functions without me, despite my encouragement for him to go. But, from the view inside my heart I saw the importance of his well-being and deeply desired to find an opening that would take us past this annual roadblock.

Discussing this particular challenge with a specialist provided an exciting alternative to explore: Cater Christmas dinner. We called a wonderful lady who had served meals for Kip's folks years before. The added expense concerned me, so I suggested to Kip that we present the meal as our Christmas gift to our family instead of giving material or monetary gifts.

The meal (for nine people) was prepared elsewhere, then brought into our home. The caterer served each guest personally, and everyone, including me, enjoyed the momentous dinner. A much appreciated part of the service included complete cleanup. We were all free to fellowship together after our meal while the caterer cleaned up. My disability prevented me from understanding the active conversation shared around the dinner table, but I drank in the blessings of the joy that was present. Smiles illuminated faces and laughter erupted. There was happiness in our home and my heart was filled with gratitude.

Eventually, exhaustion wouldn't cooperate with my efforts to ignore it, so I slipped away to a quiet room for a while. During that time the piano was brought to life again. Singing and music accompanied the celebratory spirit. Everyone was relaxed and I felt a personal victory with my determination to find a positive way to adapt. More importantly, my precious husband savoured each moment of this special time with our family. Sharing our love in this unique way was a fulfilling gift to give. And receive.

Fears are lessening, adaptations are becoming easier to accept, and new strategies are being sought. The joy of entertaining is bringing life to our home once again, particularly at Christmas, but not without an enormous amount of thought, planning, and effort. We have learned to space out our evening gatherings during this very special season, entertaining guests every Monday and Thursday evening during the month of December. The responses are rewarding. Kip and I continue to seek medical advice, and this has helped with devising plans that are plausible and workable. I must monitor my days carefully and purposefully, eliminating other fatiguing activities during this season of evening entertaining. We invite only one couple or one to two single friends per evening.

Times of fellowship are absolutely wonderful as close friends recognize the need to speak one at a time. If the men want to talk one on one, they slip into the living room and we gals visit for a while in the family room. Our guests' willingness to stick by us and learn alongside of us has enabled them to recognize the fading signs that naturally show up on my face, at which point they gracefully call it a night. Days immediately following the evening of entertainment are for renewal and recharging, permitting me to be the best I can be for our next guests. I have to say, our friends are cut from a very special cloth. They are sincere, caring, supportive, encouraging and very accepting of my limitations. In fact, one of the greatest joys to both Kip and me is the absence of focus on my disability when we fellowship together. It is a time to genuinely enjoy other folks intimately, without all the superficial chatter that often goes along with large Christmas gatherings.

Friends who have active families and fast-paced careers particularly enjoy the relaxation they find in our home. They feel tucked away from the hectic pace of the season. We share life with each other, and the gift that they bring to our home, the gift of being themselves, is the greatest gift anyone could ever hope to receive. Kip and I continually praise God Almighty for introducing us to this newfound freedom from the stress and anxiety which usually occurs during the busiest season of the year. Intriguingly, here is a new freedom discovered through the limitations of a disability.

Committed to a constant search of adaptation, we are discovering and implementing solutions which are greatly helping to ease the feelings of loneliness. It requires a lot of work, planning and determination to find solutions. It may seem easier to remain in the void that a sense of loneliness can produce, but the devastating results of that decision would generate much more than loneliness. A chasm of emptiness would eventually devour you. Turning to God the Father, baring your feelings before Him, will help to lighten the pathway of hope. For you see, as you turn your face toward Jesus, you cannot help but to witness the Light that flows from Him.

There is a growing fullness taking place in our lives as wonderful friends stop by to visit for short periods of time. We laugh, confide in each other, pray, and even sometimes sing. Emails draw hearts together despite geographical distance, enriching the soul much like sitting down for a cup of tea together. Friendships are solid, trustworthy and dependable. They are also concrete. And priceless. Just like my relationship with my Lord.

Feelings of loneliness do not flood over me as they had before, even when I am physically alone. Jesus said in John 16:32, *"Yet I am not alone, for my Father is with me."* All I need to do is whisper His name in prayer and I feel Him with me, eliminating any loneliness, like a little visit together sharing a cup of tea. And those He brings into my life are valuable jewels which sparkle and shine, dispelling any shadow of isolation.

PART FOUR

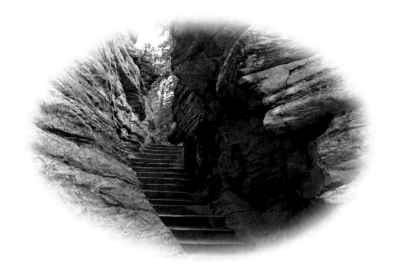

PROACTIVE FAITH

*"Now faith is being sure of what we hope for
and certain of what we do not see."*
(Hebrews 11:1)

1

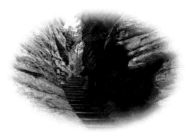

STEPS OF FAITH

KNOWLEDGE UNLOCKS THE DOOR OF UNDERSTANDING, AND understanding, if applied properly, eventually brings acceptance. In due course, true contentment will follow with the success of each task attempted and completed. Whether a task is big or small isn't of importance, really. It is the feeling of accomplishment in not giving up, and self-satisfaction ensues after persisting with a realistic physical challenge, regardless of how long it takes to complete. Our emotional consciousness of well-being strengthens each time we achieve victory over an obstacle, whatever that obstacle may be. This awareness develops as the Holy Spirit does His work deep within our hearts. Allowing His entry into that sacred place gives Him the freedom to do wonderful things. We experience it because we have allowed unbridled access to our hearts.

Looking back, I can clearly see God's provision for me each moment of each day. He was right there by my side through that entire tragedy as it transpired. My family physician had just arrived on duty in the emergency room when I came in by ambulance. This gave my husband *some* sense of peace, as he trusted our doctor completely. I believe the Lord knew how much Kip needed that reassurance.

We also experienced excellent care within the medical field from the onset. I experienced it personally being the one with the disability, and my husband experienced it as the one who was committed to stay by my side. Life as I had known it for forty-one years had become fragmented, yet our loving God provided an abundance of knowledgeable, caring and compassionate professionals who educated us, encouraged us, and committed to support us through the long term. Proverbs 15:22 says, *"Plans fail for lack of counsel, but with many advisers they succeed."* Through knowledge and understanding, I found hope in answers that eased my uncertainty of the life-altering changes taking place.

Lessons in life are enormously valuable. Lessons, even on the most challenging training ground, will always provide opportunity for personal growth. The only time a lesson would threaten to stunt our growth would be if we chose to keep our eyes on the difficulty of the challenge that lies ahead without lifting our heads toward the Light— toward Almighty God for strength, guidance and courage.

One of the greatest lessons I have discovered is the value of reaching out with a willingness to seek support from professionals, both medically and spiritually. Shortly after being diagnosed with a permanent brain injury, I was encouraged to contact a local psychologist who held a special professional interest in brain-injured persons. I stewed for days, looking at her phone number, wondering if I should call. The frustrations had placed me in a battle of daily unknowns and I found myself wandering aimlessly in very unfamiliar territory.

My entire life I had never needed to speak with a psychologist, and pride was the invisible arm that pulled me away each time I went to call her. Finally, one day I pushed that invisible arm aside, realizing I would remain in this battle without any kind of armour against the inevitable difficulties that were ahead if I didn't call her. I needed knowledge from someone who could help me understand how to proceed in life, instead of receding. What a blessing she turned out to be! She was kind, nonjudgmental, and positive, and she offered tremendous encouragement. I could share things with her in total confidence. Through that process I found answers to questions I was afraid to ask anyone else due to fears of being viewed as "incompetent."

It's not only okay to ask many, many questions, but asking those questions is critical to taking positive steps forward. Taking that risk of vulnerability is indicative of a spirit that yearns to move forward. Crucial, however, is the process of seeking out qualified advisors, and some sifting is needed before accessing true professional experts who can give adequate and appropriate counsel.

Accepting that this disability is permanent has definitely been taking time. It will continue to take time and it will continue to test me. Growing in the understanding of my disability and learning to be patient with my limitations often seems to progress much slower than I would like, but I am determined to advance from baby steps to toddler steps as I pursue success. A lifetime of change is on the path before me. Alterations and adjustments will forever vary as circumstances impose new challenges. Medications I take will be constantly monitored, as some work well while others have not. The individual activities I encounter each day largely determine what I can and cannot do. Progression involves scrutiny, and decision-making will result from a myriad of factors.

I believe God gives each one of us a spirit of courage. He also gives us strength to climb whatever mountains appear before us in our lives. He considers our personal and individual limitations, and provides absolutely everything we need to overcome obstacles. He is more than capable to help us each day. And if tomorrow brings a more difficult challenge, then our Lord's provision will be more abundant.

Each obstacle is very different. Life does not stand still. Having experienced excursions to various mountain summits in the magnificent Canadian Rockies, I can confidently testify that a true high envelops your entire being as you drink in the breathtaking, all-encompassing beauty. You cannot comprehend the resplendent view at the summit from the valleys and forests below. It is absolutely impossible.

I liken this literal experience to the figurative mountains in our lives. When we begin our climb we feel fresh, sure-footed, assertive and driven.

As the pathway becomes more difficult, apprehension begins to trickle in. We look up, seeing only obstacles to overcome, such as trees, cliffs, boulders, or wide streams. Climbing higher we encounter more trees, cliffs, boulders and streams, and our energy reserve starts to wane. From a distance this mountain had seemed much smaller, convincing us it was worth the challenge. Now, our limited vision may cause doubt as to whether we should proceed any further. We don't see very far in front of us, and at some point weariness challenges our strength and our spirit of determination. We may even begin to question whether the view from the top of the mountain is even worth the climb to get there.

Finally, the summit is gloriously exposed and we become entranced by the grandeur of the magnificence all around. Various shades of green in the trees contrast the gray, jagged cliffs of rock, some covered with puffs of pure white snow. Emerald streams flow from glaciers, making sweet mountain music which fills our senses and renews our soul. We feel alive! Doubt no longer exists. Those former "obstacles" take on a different form, appearing magnificent and worthy of their placement. We realize that those challenging obstacles along the way to the top were instrumental in the design and creation of this magnificent view. Every single encounter was simply part of the process to grow us, to stretch us to a higher level of personal achievement. Others will never experience this level of victory unless they pursue their own personal climb to the top, with obstacles of their own to overcome.

So it is with the mountains which rise before us in our lives, daily hurdles that challenge our whole being. Obstacles that test our endurance, forcing us to question whether we should carry on. Yet, what awaits? Choosing to go back, you may feel defeat and loss of self-esteem. Internal questions may nip at you: "What if I had kept going?" Pressing onward with a hope-driven persistence, however, will result in a stronger spirit sweetened by the taste of personal victory! And that is worth the daily climb. Many times, rivers of questions asking "Why, why, why?" are answered as we proceed through the years ahead. Steps taken in faith, regardless of the inability to see the outcome, encourage us to place our trust in the promise of what lies ahead. Understanding evolves as we confront, and overcome, individual obstacles. It is then we can stand at the top of a particular mountain in life, relishing the magnificent view, thankful, ever so thankful we didn't turn back. We have grown. Each victory attained produces growth, and growth produces a positively changed life.

We may hear from others tales of spectacular beauty discovered on the summit of a mountain. Yet we can never fully grasp understanding of their emotions until we experience it ourselves. Our own personal experiences and growth will differ vastly from others'. We are all unique, laying claim to individual strengths, weaknesses, and methods of strategy. But the end result of personal growth and victory will be just as exuberant as another's, and healthy self-esteem will take root and flourish.

We need to continually place our faith and trust in God our Father. He is our infallible Guide and it is only He who knows the pathway which leads to the fulfillment of His purpose. Our loving Father leads us one step at a time. We must place absolute faith and trust in Him, even though we may not see what lies ahead. He knows the view from the top. He alone knows what we need to learn and what must be overcome so we can experience our own personal victories. Proverbs 3:5 says, *"Trust in the LORD with all your heart and lean not on your own understanding."* My own understanding may whisper to me that I cannot overcome, that something is impossible to do or to do well. Almighty God wants me to trust Him with all of my heart. He does not simply want me to just overcome obstacles, battles, uncertainties and challenges. He desires that I *thrive* in this gift of life He has intimately chosen for me. He wants me to experience much more than just simple existence. He wants me to experience abundant life found only through His Son, Jesus Christ.

God is our eternal Guide. It is true that personal accomplishments and victories are important for maintaining healthy self-esteem, yet it is only through Him that we are able to claim those victories. As we journey along this pathway of life, our faithful and trustworthy Heavenly Guide is truly the One Who deserves all the glory. He will never take us to a place where He is not in complete control. It is He Who remains faithful to directing our uncertain steps.

2

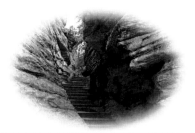

ACCEPTANCE

LEARNING TO ACCEPT THE CHANGES I WAS HAVING TO MAKE, AND WOULD have to continue to make, was going to take time. It also meant being patient for answers to unfold. Time, I suddenly had an abundance of. Patience … well, I needed to concentrate heavily on that part. Early on in my disability, I placed unrealistic expectations on myself that caused frustration and many tears. I just knew that if I tried hard enough, I would be able to overcome these limitations and my life would be "normal" again. Before the accident, I had so much responsibility and I greatly enjoyed the challenges. Kip and I knew each other extremely well, and he had depended on my skills and contributions both at work and at home.

Our business had grown to corporation status and the future was exciting. Without warning, I was unable to fulfill my role as a business partner. His business partner. The business began to suffer tremendously and we had to find workable solutions—quickly. Uncertainty, and out-of-town medical appointments, produced such upheaval in 2002 and 2003 that we almost lost our business. I was no longer able to multi-task, my short-term memory was impaired, noise was unbearable from the main street, and various conversations were scrambled. I couldn't make decisions. I found myself lost trying to follow instructions regarding new applications, and extreme fatigue forced me to immediately lie down in the warehouse or in the car (depending on the weather), notwithstanding the fact I was often trying to work with a client at the time.

Confronted daily with the fact that many areas of our lives were greatly suffering, we had to find solid solutions. It was painfully obvious I could no longer remain active in our boutique. Losing the career I loved so much was very difficult to accept. I deeply missed interaction with clients, along with the rewarding hum of activity in the boutique. Most months, we worked with approximately sixty clients. Beyond my administrative work, I had also baked muffins or buns to give to clients as a thank-you for their business. It was a unique way in which we did business, and we had built a mini kitchen within the boutique to allow me to do this. We were grateful for each and every client that came through the door and we wanted them to know that, in a personal way.

Kip was also adversely affected by this disability. He lost his partner in a growing business and was doing everything he could to help manage household necessities when he wasn't at the boutique. My disability enormously affected the amount of work I could do, even at home. Taking three times longer to accomplish everything, my productivity was extremely limited. I saw his exhaustion and wanted desperately to alleviate it. But I couldn't reverse what had happened. I felt so inadequate.

The gift of change was sitting on my doorstep. I tripped over it each time I fought against this disability. I needed to decide whether to let it sit there unopened, throw away the opportunities tucked inside, or open the gift, allowing it to positively influence my life. Bruised with frustration, I finally chose to pick it up. Before opening it, I needed to acknowledge exactly what position I was in now. What did I know, and what did I not know. Most importantly, what did I need to learn?

The facts were before me. My brain was no longer functioning the way it used to and I was going to have to accept that. I had knowledge of my disability. Mild Traumatic Brain Injury had set up house, permanently. It didn't matter how hard I tried, I now knew I could not replace what had been lost. I had begun to recognize the importance of surrendering guilt, often resulting from my perceived inadequacies, to God. Through God's grace and faithfulness, I began to consciously push aside the temptation to step back into my old shoes. Counselling from my physician and other professionals gave me tremendous support and encouragement as I began to identify my areas of limitation, seeking proactive ways to adapt.

This process was deliberate and confrontational. Instead of turning around to see what I was leaving behind, I made a commitment to look straight ahead at the challenge before me. I had to remind myself every single time that I must not look at the whole battlefield, only the battle that was directly in front of me at that particular time. It was time to straighten my armour. It was time to move forward.

I began to accept that I would never be able to contribute to our business as I had previously done. This, of course, was one of the biggest areas of difficulty for me to accept. Yet it was not just I who had to deal with that realization. Kip had to accept it as well. While in a meeting with one specialist, Kip had mentioned that I was his "right arm" in business. Stunning both of us, the specialist declared sternly, "Wrong! She will *never* be your right arm again and you've got to accept that! For her sake and yours!" Taken off guard, we opened the gates of denial, releasing tears as the specialist brought the harsh truth to the forefront. He was not one to pussy-foot around the truth, truth based on fact. He knew what he saw. Forcing us to come face to face with the reality that I would never physically participate in the boutique anymore seemed ruthless at first. Yet he was there to help us move forward. With clearer vision, both Kip and I were able to map out a much wiser approach to the challenges ahead. As arduous as this advisor was, he was one of the best we had, and we knew he was on our side.

My physician cautioned me that repetitive focus on doing the impossible would constantly deprive me of the satisfaction and contentment I could have in other areas of my life. He was absolutely right. I carefully considered what he said and this helped me take a huge step forward. I wanted life, abundant life. I did not want to continue living a life that was full of chaos, frustration and chronic failure.

When God closes one door, He always opens another. It was my responsibility to recognize that. He stayed right beside me when I kept trying to re-open the door of my past. He patiently waited, time and time again, allowing me to discover the futile pursuit of what used to be. Only I could close that door forever. I had to make a conscious decision to look for the new, open door I was to go through. Placing my feet into unfamiliar territory would require complete trust in Him. Entering the unknown can be unsettling, but I knew I could trust the One Who would take my hand. He would guide me, but it I had to be ready to accept His guidance. He patiently waited until I was ready. Finally I closed the old door and reached out in faith for His hand. It was right there.

God's Word was my map. Never being one to sit back and let life go by, I wasn't going to let that happen now. But I needed direction, or more importantly, redirection. I had been identifying my personal worth with the things I did. If I couldn't work, entertain or manage my home, what was I really contributing? How would others view me? Would I be disappointing God? Would I be letting Kip down? What on earth was my purpose if I couldn't do these "simple" things? As I carefully considered these questions, then searched for the answers in God's Word, life started to take on new meaning. Hebrews 12:2 says, *"Let us fix our eyes on Jesus, the author and perfecter of our faith."* I knew He had allowed these changes, but I needed to acknowledge that I couldn't recognize His will for my life. Looking backward prevented me from seeing the possibilities that lay ahead. Turning away from Jesus, I had kept trying to rely on myself. Without Him, failure was inevitable.

I am grateful Jesus accepts me just as I am. Sometimes I am amazed at how incredibly patient He is with me. He wants me to recognize and use the gifts I still have and He expects me to use wisdom as I search for His will. Not all has been lost. God has been moulding me since the day I was born. The first forty-one years were exactly as He had planned. He doesn't want me to throw that all away. In fact, He wants to grow me beyond the place I was at in 2001. That's a staggering thought, considering that I now have a permanent brain injury! He has chosen to redirect my life. I need to understand and accept that, because when He's in control exciting things will happen. Trying to turn back the clock to a familiar, comfortable place was getting me into trouble. He has given me new gifts, leaving many of my former gifts intact. In fact, learning to identify the new gifts He's introducing is stirring an excitement for life I thought had been lost. He invites and challenges me to explore each one, and He expects me to use them for His glory.

I recently read this inspiring phrase: *To dream of the person you used to be is to waste the person you are.* Acceptance is not resignation or giving up hope. It is embracing change with clear recognition of moving forward. Recognition of what has moulded and shaped me becomes evident, but further down the pathway, carefully chosen gifts wait to be opened. Those gifts of change are unwrapped slowly, gently encouraging the exploration of each viable opportunity. Acceptance of change produces a healthy confidence. My purpose in life is not to search out the easy road for my own gratification. My role and purpose in life is to live for Christ. The clearer my focus on what God's Word says, the clearer my life's purpose will become.

Acceptance of challenges strengthens me. Overcoming hurdles replaces frustration with anticipation, and I obtain satisfaction through successful problem-solving. I conquer challenges through direct reliance on Christ and the power of the Holy Spirit. When I see how my relationship with Christ produces positive results, acceptance of my disability comes much easier. I will continue to fall short of fulfilling the many plans I have, but what is so awesome is that God usually brings new plans into the picture I didn't even think of—better plans. At times, He replaces my plans with His plans to ensure the work gets done that He intends for me to do. Proverbs 16:9 affirms this: *"In his heart a man plans his course, but the LORD determines his steps."* It's very important for me to make plans and have dreams. God did not create me to be a puppet. He expects me to be proactive in this walk with Him. However, I must lift those plans and dreams up to Him for His divine approval in order to experience complete freedom of abundant living.

I must focus on doing my best, continually looking for and finding ways to adapt, accepting the limitations I have. James 1:22–25 says,

*Do not merely **listen** to the word, and so deceive yourselves. **Do** what it says. Anyone who listens to the word but does not do what it says is like a man who looks at his face in a mirror and, after looking at himself, goes away and immediately forgets what he looks like. But the man who looks intently into the perfect law that gives freedom, and continues to do this, not forgetting what he has heard, but doing it—he will be blessed in what he does.* (Emphasis mine)

At one point, I was the person looking into the mirror, wondering who on earth I was. I was talking with God, but it was I who was doing all the talking without stopping to listen to what God needed to tell me. True, restorative communion with Him is never a one-way street.

I want God's blessing in everything I do. I want freedom in Christ. Acceptance says no to the whispers of Satan as he tries to turn my heart away from Christ to focus on myself, my weaknesses and the limitations of my disability. He will endlessly try to make me feel like a failure. But God promises that His gifts and promises are good and perfect. James 1:16–17 says, *"Don't be deceived, my dear brothers. Every good and perfect gift is from above, coming down from the Father of the heavenly lights, who does not change like shifting shadows."* Circumstances will change, people will change, life will change. But God, our Almighty Heavenly Father, will never change.

Continual acceptance of who I am in Him gives my life consistency and a healthy sense of self-worth. Nothing could be more rewarding than accepting and applying His "good and perfect gifts" daily. Browning once wrote, "God's gifts put man's best dreams to shame."[1] How foolish to leave His gifts unopened! How foolish to think my dreams can bring more joy to life than His! Sometimes I can hardly contain the freedom I'm discovering in His everlasting faithfulness.

Beyond this internal acceptance are the cherished jewels of relationships that will allow nothing to come between them. Acceptance from beyond myself. Although everyone struggles with the changes that

---

[1] Browning, Elizabeth Barrett, Sonnets from the Portugese XXVI I Lived with Visions for my Company Closing Line

a recently acquired disability will bring, there are those who will stand "closer than a brother." Support, acceptance and encouragement from friends and family members who choose to really desire understanding of the disability greatly contribute to the success and consistency of the journey. Humour and love seem to cover any idiosyncrasies from the past that could threaten new growth.

Dinner is often brought, bought or cooked by others at our home when someone wants to get together for a meal. It has become "normal" to celebrate meals together this way, allowing me to enjoy a couple of hours of fellowship with a small group of three or four in total. Family and friends automatically don headsets for the television. Outside yard work with noisy tools "boys" enjoy is done early in the morning, when my medication is most effective and I'm freshest. "Put in your ear plugs, Kath!" This is often called out if a noisy activity is going to take place (such as using the chainsaw or leaf blower). Pinecones are thrown against my office window, a secret code alerting me to the fact that someone outside needs to talk to me (we chose not to have a doorbell). Girlfriends call or drop by in the morning for a visit. Offers to take my car in for a tune-up on a rainy day, or requests to pick up some items at the store are "No problem." Thoughtful suggestions and reminders come readily when I forget certain things that need to be done. The list goes on.

When tragedy first strikes, confusion filters into everyone involved. But as time passes, discovering new ways to get the most out of life become a new norm. Unfamiliarity begins to turn into a new and comfortable familiarity. As years pass, memories of how certain things used to be become foggy, thus providing easier acceptance of how things are done now. The message which echoes from all who are my faithful cheerleaders is this: "You mean more to me than just the things you can do. We'll figure it out together." That's true friendship and love! That's unconditional acceptance! And it produces a deep, deep desire to continue to press forward.

3

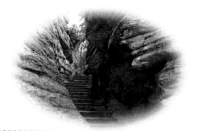

Choices

A VERY CONSEQUENTIAL MOVE IN *MY* MIND WAS WHEN KIP AND I DECIDED to seek professional Christian counsel. The Bible instructs us to seek counsel. Proverbs 13:10 says, *"But wisdom is found in those who take advice."* Proverbs 15:22 also instructs, *"Plans fail for lack of counsel, but with many advisers they succeed."* God had previously led us to professional counsel, providing specifically educated medical advisors. Their assessments and knowledge regarding the effects of my brain injury helped enormously in my understanding of what was taking place within my brain and body, both emotionally and physically. However, the next phase found my soul yearning for spiritual guidance, particularly in certain areas.

Initially, I needed to identify what my situation was in order to understand how to cope with it. Much of my focus had been on the medical side of the changes within me, and this had taken priority. My relationship with the Lord was deepening, yet hurdles remained which

I couldn't go over, under, around or through. Some were visible, some were not.

Seeking out a professional Christian counsellor challenged my courage. I felt very vulnerable knowing discussions would be elevated to a spiritual level. How I thank God for His provision of the counsellor we decided to meet with! As I sought spiritual wisdom and guidance during one-on-one sessions with him, those hurdles became less menacing. I was advised to focus on what God expects of me. I was challenged to reach deep within my heart for answers to that. I was also urged to evaluate my personal walk with the Lord, both prior to the accident and during its aftermath.

This was an arduous process, as blotches and stains show up when exposed to the Light. I am a sinner. Daily. Voluntarily at times and involuntarily at others. Old stains are immediately wiped clean the moment I seek forgiveness, but fresh new stains stand out shamelessly. Through tears of repentance, I was once again cleansed by the blood of the Lamb. This necessary cleansing opened the way to enormous freedom. Because of the blood of Jesus Christ, the slate was clean once again. Shrouded truths slowly became more visible. God does not expose all truths at one time; He gives them within His perfect agenda. He knows we can only absorb so much, so He is careful and tenderly guides His children one step at a time.

I became more astute toward the value of choices. Each decision made is a healthy choice or an unhealthy one, but is completely mine to make. I had been struggling enormously, feeling as though I was losing sight of who I was. I needed to reach for God's hand, allowing Him to rescue me from drowning in a sea of turmoil. I wanted to once again experience His gift of abundant life.

Important choices were before me. I could choose to focus on the uncertainty each day would bring, thus continuing down a road leading to unhappiness and an unfulfilled life. I could choose to withdraw from life, angry and bitter at God for allowing this to happen to me. Or I could choose to acknowledge my worth in Christ's eyes, which held much greater promise for the potential to experience a lifetime of adventure, step by step, day by day. I could choose to open my eyes to the hope of a new journey, placing my will aside, enticed by the opportunity to know God's will and purpose for this imperfect vessel. With committed resolve, I chose adventure.

Seeking God's guidance and listening to His precious voice definitely increases the odds for success, from God's point of view. The daily choice to read God's Word, along with a yearning to apply what I read to my life, took time. Reading was not a strong point anymore (a big disappointment for me). My speed was impaired greatly, so I achieved understanding more slowly as I tried to comprehend what I was reading. Sentences often wove in and out of each other. Yet, I was hungry to know what God had planned for me. Discipline on my part was essential. It was the only way I could succeed. One day at a time, I would pick up my beloved Bible and read a small portion, using a blank piece of paper to guide my eyes in the proper direction. Then, I would pray. God is so truly personal. Because the Bible is written in verses and chapters, I found myself picking it up more frequently. Communing with this amazing, loving God through His Holy Living Word cannot be described. It must be experienced. On a daily basis.

Committed to daily devotions, Kip and I felt more confident in confronting the enormous tasks before us. Spending time with the Lord doesn't eliminate the battles, but it makes an enormous difference as to the plan of attack. It also clarifies Who our Leader is. Our humanness in the form of feelings and emotions still intrudes. Answers don't always come readily. Then again, answers may come readily, but they might be completely different from what we anticipated. The difference is found in the comfort of knowing that God is in complete control, regardless of the severity of the situation at hand. My disability was the situation at hand. It had permanence and important decisions needed to be made.

Our concern over how we would continue to operate our business was at the forefront of our thoughts. It was our livelihood, therefore it was necessary to evaluate the reality of the situation. We needed to take stock of the entire scope of circumstances in order to correctly assess what decisions needed to be made. We had both worked incredibly hard to build our business to where it was, and we almost lost it in 2002 and 2003, due to accident-related issues. Our only source of income, the serious risk of losing it remained worrisome. During this time, I underwent intense testing by a professional vocational specialist who assessed my ability to work successfully in a competitive workforce. Was the potential there for me to return to my work and my career one day? Was there another line of work available to me for continued employment? Not only for financial reasons, but also for the health and well-being of my self-esteem. Along with my husband, I had operated a successful, thriving business and it was a vital part of my life. My skills were valuable and strong. It was important to me and it gave my life direction and focus.

After several assessments and examinations, the vocational assessor concluded that I would not be able to function adequately in the conventional workplace again. Due to many factors relating to my brain injury, it was unfeasible for me to re-enter the marketplace of employment competitively. My ability to process information was too slow, and my inability to multi-task or shut out distractions was a definite impairment.

This was very difficult to absorb. I had always enjoyed working, having taken on my first job at a very young age as a page (filing books away) in the City of Calgary Public Library. Fatigue blanketed over me following the days of testing, and my heart was discouraged. I was trying so hard to trust God. I was trying so hard to truly believe He was in control. There *were* times of peace and of certainty. There were also times when my faith was severely shaken. Kip and I did experience God's Presence, but my heart spiraled downward as if on a rollercoaster when another facet of discouragement presented itself, as it did with the results of the vocational testing. That familiar battle with guilt threatened to wage war inside of me when again I was told I could not operate our business with my husband as we had for years. What would we do? How would we manage financially?

The tests basically confirmed what I already knew but was unsuccessfully trying to disguise. I was very aware of the impossibility to function as needed in a professional environment. Now clinically affirmed, my brain injury limitations would prevent me from further pursuing the career I loved. Harsh reality glowered back at me—at us. More apparent than ever was the fact that we had to find solutions quickly.

Scrambling to save our business, Kip and I set aside some time for an emergency meeting to review where we were at. Operating a business of your own, particularly a successful business, requires much more than eight-hour shifts five days per week. You are also aware that your staff depend on you for their jobs. More lives were involved than just ours. We were faced with two options. The first was to give up, lose it all, having the doors closed for us. The second option was to unearth workable solutions to save our business. A decision to shut down the shop would necessitate Kip to find a new job. The consideration of that decision was not long-lived, as Kip has a special God-given gift for interior design. He also excels in business management, having many years of experience to his credit. Most of all, he loved his work and our boutique.

That first assessment revealed that the critical issue needing to be assessed was not Kip's position, but mine. With all cards laid on the table, the administrative component of the business was the area of most concern. If we acquired clerical help and additional staff to oversee the shop, Kip could do his job. We believed this decision would enable business to get back on track again. Naming the primary hurdle blocking our path gave us a more defined idea of what we needed to tackle first. Acceptance on my part would definitely make the changes easier.

We had invited our Heavenly Father to chair the meeting. After all, everything we have is His. We have always recognized His ownership, however we were the ones called to manage that which He had blessed us with. Sure we had dreams and goals for the business, and we knew God always listened attentively when we shared those with Him. But His purpose always yields the greatest fruit. As Proverbs 19:21 says, *"Many are the plans in a man's heart, but it is the LORD'S purpose that prevails."* We sought God's wisdom and direction. We tried to listen prudently to His instructions. We wanted His will to prevail.

This important management meeting opened doors to some key choices. Cautiously allowing hope to seep into our hearts, we followed God's leading to hire additional staff. This was an enormous step of faith as we put complete trust in God. We felt sure of His direction, but did not know where the finances would come from to support this kind of staff. Due to out-of-town assessments, Kip's absence forced spurts of temporary closure of the boutique. We were struggling just to keep the business afloat. Yet we had consulted with our Lord and our job was to trust Him as we ventured forward in obedience. We hired one part-time employee at first, subsequently hiring a full-time employee within the following year. We also made the choice to manage our business differently, fully recognizing I could no longer work at the boutique.

God often works through other people. We sought guidance and help from others we trusted. In retrospect, God's provision was clearly evident as we had to reach out for increased assistance from professionals we had been working with for years. I believe our initial prudent choices of those professionals were directed by the Lord, as He had known well in advance this life-altering change was going to take place, and when. The development of strong professional relationships prior to the accident created a solid foundation of knowledge and familiarity with the way we ran our business. Many of my responsibilities were reassigned to people we had worked closely with for years, those who knew our stalwart expectations for the business. Our accountant remained by our side through every step of difficulty experienced within the business. She also cheered alongside of us as victories replaced what could have been unbearable failure. Beyond that, she is a woman of high caliber, and a friend I enormously respect and cherish. Witnessing God's hand at work through that whole process is beyond adequate description. He is more than worthy of our trust, to that we can passionately attest. It was yet another validation of our Father's loyal faithfulness to His children when they call upon His name.

I knew beyond any shadow of a doubt that I wanted to remain involved with the business, but I didn't know how. Before me was another crossroad, yet an interesting one to explore. Hence began my investigation into seeking out possibilities. I had been striving hard to accept the reality of not being able to work in a conventional business environment because of noise factors, distractions, and slower speed of processing information. However, my spirit was a lot more resistant to admitting that I couldn't work at all! God had given me certain strengths and He had chosen to leave my level of reasoning intact. After all, I had been reassured I was still "smart." What then were my options?

Determined to remain an active although somewhat silent business partner, I decided to try to work from home. This solution offered a great deal of encouragement for me as the feasibility to control my surroundings was promising. An Occupational Therapist assessed our home. She explained how and why I needed to do certain things and she determined which room would be suitable to work in. She did not want my office on the beach side of our home, as she felt the distractions would hamper my productivity. She was absolutely right. Her ability to make sound decisions that would work in my favour was invaluable. This eliminated a lot of stress and frustration for me. I still think of her often, especially when the beach side is busy and I am still able to work quietly and productively in the room she appointed.

I found myself being able to work successfully at my own pace. I no longer had the pressures of instantaneous decision-making which was required on a regular basis at the boutique. The revolving door of activity buzzing around in the flurry of a busy boutique was eliminated. Due to the fact that my ability to process information takes three times longer than normal, this modification was significant.

Over a period of time, in the quietness of my office I gained a strong sense of what tasks were too overwhelming and what tasks were manageable. Each time I had to relinquish a specific task, I naturally felt some loss. Step by step, the choice to continue to work in a modified environment slowly replaced discouragement as I began to experience healthier, less stressful days. Delegation became more comfortable. Satisfaction of my accomplishments became more prevalent and a sense of fulfillment kept the tears of discouragement away, producing a smile at the end of the day. Gradually weeding through my strengths and weaknesses had minimized direct involvement, however I still enjoyed interaction with staff and other professionals on a regular basis. There was just one area of persistent difficulty.

Creating advertisements was the one task I was determined to hang onto. It was my baby. I took great pride in the area of advertising, having created our ads every second week for twelve years. They were very effective. My skills were acknowledged locally and we were rewarded with great sales. The results and recognition had been personally satisfying. After the accident, it became a struggle for me. Every second week, I became extremely overwhelmed by the responsibility. Due to my reduced cognitive speed, I spent countless hours putting an ad together to meet the deadline. Once submitted and put into ad form, it was returned for approval. I was slower at processing, but still sharp regarding accuracy. Sometimes it would take two or three proofs to perfect it. Managing the advertising while multi-tasking other administrative duties had been the norm for me. I had once thrived at this pace, but that was not possible anymore. Through God's gentle nudging, I made the choice to train a staff member to assume the responsibility.

A valued and trusted colleague of mine often said to me, "No one is beyond replacement in the professional world, Kath. There are many others just waiting in the wings to step into the shoes of another." This was meant to encourage me, and it did when making critical staffing decisions. Pondering her words, I had to face the reality that someone else could do a great job with the ads. After training and guidance, we delegated my advertising responsibility to another and yes, the job was well done. My employee was eager to learn and she always ran them by me before sending them off to print.

God is very clear when He lets us know it's time to let go. I hung onto the advertising work with great tenacity, telling God (and my hubby) that this was the last area defining my career. I wasn't going to give it up, too. Yet every two weeks I was exceedingly tired, fully aware that this area was draining me. Well, when you refuse to accept what the Lord is telling you, He will humble your heart. Surrendering to His nudging, I finally resolved to let go and, "waiting in the wings" was a qualified gal who was eager to learn from me. God enabled me to share my knowledge with another. Privately I mused, "Was this a loss or has it perhaps been a gift, enabling someone else to grow?"

The professional team we work with have encouraged me to let go of that which I can no longer do. They are enormously supportive of me in the tasks I still do, and all of them continue to respect me as a professional woman and business owner. We correspond via email, with the occasional phone call. We hold meetings early in the morning in quiet boardrooms away from office activity. Sales reps involved with our business for years often come out to our home to visit with me and involve me in the updates of their products. We've even had training seminars at home, allowing me to slip away when I need to.

The tremendous support and encouragement of these wonderful professionals, along with enormous modifications produced by a determined spirit to move forward, has enabled me to continue to work. Learning of these adaptations, the vocational assessor said, "Had you not owned your own business to make appropriate modifications in, and had you not been determined to experiment with the possibilities of failure or success, the options to return to the working world would be diminutive, *if* there were any at all." He was pleased that the opportunity to valuably contribute to our business was still accessible to me, no matter how minimal my involvement. He felt it was extremely important to my progress and growth. His support and exhortation certainly strengthened my resolve to search the depth of my spirit when challenged with perceived "impossibilities." Once again, God's divine planning years ago, guiding and leading us through the operation of our business, allowed positive solutions to an unforeseen and otherwise grim situation.

The business is thriving once again, and although there will always be continual changes, my husband and I enjoy our partnership afresh. He continues to involve me in critical decisions, and I still confer with professionals who have remained steadfast through the hornet's nest of uncertainty. Every night, Kip and I sit together at the dinner table and recap our day's events. This keeps me in the loop and I am aware of everything that takes place at the boutique.

No, this was not the professional pathway I was expecting. This new pathway has led to dynamic changes in my life professionally; however, Kip and I have the privilege of viewing the corporate world from a much different perspective than most. We have experienced ongoing corporate integrity, wisdom, respect, encouragement, support and kindness which have greatly assisted us in the necessary changes needing to take place. In today's society, particularly in the corporate world, these qualities are rare. We never take for granted the professionals assisting us as we continue to proceed with the business God has placed in our care.

God gave us this business opportunity many years ago, and we sought to honour Him in every facet. My disability thrust us onto a very bumpy road occupationally. Although my direct input is very restricted, I am still employed, working within my capabilities to do a job that is satisfying. Delightfully, the voice of my physician echoes in my heart, "Good news, Kathie. You are still smart." By the grace of God, my intelligence level and ability to reason had not been damaged. Critical choices needing to be made were within my professional realm, largely due to corporate support, Kip's support, and a God-given spirit of determination. I am learning to be content with my modified and ever-changing professional role.

Choices determining day-to-day activities needed to be addressed as well. Cleaning help at home was required weekly instead of bi-weekly. Grocery shopping, a task which involves timely decision-making and large amounts of activity, was almost unbearable for me. Music, announcements, searching for items, conversations and fast-paced checkouts drained every ounce of energy from me, resulting in confusion when it was time to pay for the groceries.

I tried to find different ways and times to do this task, but the end result was always the same. The task was overwhelming. Kip would often pick up items after he was finished work, but we still needed bigger grocery shops every so often. This area of help was more difficult to attain. For a brief period, a locally owned grocery store did their best to help out. I faxed the grocery list to them, and an employee would pick out the groceries I requested. At the end of the day, Kip would drive to the store to pick them up. The owner was very kind and his thoughtfulness meant a great deal to us. Unfortunately, this alternative didn't work out, as some items requested weren't included, and items I didn't request (and couldn't use) were in the bags. This got to be expensive, and Kip couldn't go back and forth all the time trying to get the right products. It just depended on which employee did the physical shopping for me. The owner's intent was so sincere, but the differences between my order and what we received was becoming too costly.

Kip sought help through other sources but made no headway. This was disappointing and discouraging, as we had been involved with a couple of these organizations for years, one in particular. Aware of our unproductive search, a close friend of mine offered to get our groceries every second week, thus easing pressure and fatigue in that area. Extra help was also required to manage bigger household tasks such as cleaning out the fridge, sorting through the pantry, wiping down blinds and ironing. Mopping the patterned floor and ironing patterned items initiated a nauseous stomach and dizziness, forcing me to lie down for several moments until it subsided. It was a strange feeling. These things are done monthly now.

God, in His faithfulness, had provided a beautiful Christian woman to help with cleaning our home periodically long before the accident. She willingly stepped into areas I found most difficult. She has been an enormous blessing in our lives, and our friendship has deepened significantly through our bond in Christ. She has remained by my side, smoothing the way to much easier days through her incredible insight. She knew the old me and she knows the new me very, very well. Her thoughtfulness cannot be matched. She allows me room to attempt things on my own, but she also recognizes signs of needing help. Humour is a constant as we giggle and laugh over the silliest things. She is a true joy. Her friendship is a treasured gift in my life.

We have had to make many other choices and decisions, some turning out better than others. And as I progress through each day, more decisions will need to be made. God's guidance is enabling me to make necessary changes in order to produce satisfactory results as I figure out what works and what doesn't.

Choices are always there for the choosing. If some do not work out (and some won't), that's okay. Learning to accept that takes time. It also requires a great deal of patience to wait out the results of a decision made. But there would be greater failure in not even trying to find a solution. Any effort to accomplish something, regardless of the inability to know if it is going to be successful, creates growth. Learning from mistakes develops our character and (hopefully) prevents us from going a second round of bad decision-making in that same type of situation. The next time we will be wiser and our efforts just might produce success.

Reaching out to others for assistance creates an incredible opportunity for friendship. It also provides peace of mind, knowing something important is taken care of, and taken care of well. I'm learning it is not a sign of weakness, but rather of strength, as I surrender these and future tasks with the realization that God has given special gifts to others who are more than willing to share them with me. In return, I have the opportunity to experience kindheartedness which allows me to progress successfully with the tasks I am able to do. Working through this process has allowed me to discover hidden abilities which were longing to be exposed.

I will persist in seeking God's guidance as I prudently walk along this new pathway. I deeply desire to move forward, contributing to life in a positive way using my God-given talents, gifts and personality. I believe God is introducing new avenues He wants me to explore. I am excited about the opportunity to open new doors with the freedom God gives to analyze the list of choices before me. I must not glance back to what has been lost. Rather, I must face forward with anticipation for the surprises that wait ahead.

Choices are wonderful gifts. They offer an upside to every trial in life. They are available in abundance, waiting to be unwrapped and discovered, all the while shaping and moulding our character and personalities.

I know He wants to grow me, and I *want* to be grown.

4

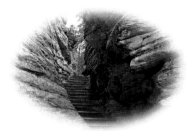

RETRAINING

THERE ARE SO MANY FACETS TO A BRAIN INJURY OF WHICH THE MAJORITY of society isn't aware. I received a lot of advice on how to cope with it, how to "work my way through it," and how to "overcome it." What most people don't realize is that you can't will yourself to "get better." In the early stages of diagnosis, I grabbed every single piece of advice that came my way, trying to apply it to my chaotic life. I did not realize at the time that doing so was creating even more chaos in an already unfamiliar world. As a result, I failed time and time again to return to my safe, reliable and comfortable way of living.

Meeting with one specialist in particular shed some much needed light upon the maze of misunderstanding and misconception. He was a specialist in the field of head trauma injury. He was also a well-renowned psychiatrist, and frequently spoke at brain injury conventions. He told me I would have to work really hard to recognize important signals alerting me to specific ways in which my brain would retrain me. I had to accept that I could not ever retrain my brain. The option to retrain my brain was not even feasible.

He proceeded further. First, I had to surrender my former way of living. This was the only possible route toward producing healthy, successful alternatives for the future. I needed to consider and accept the facts as they were, consciously and frequently pushing emotions and frustrations aside. Of particular importance was the process of learning to discern between well-meaning advice and educated advice. There would be folks who sincerely meant well but didn't have any medical knowledge about brain injuries. Additionally, advice would come from professionals who had the background of knowledge and experience to substantiate their advice. Their advice would have the same positive focus as I did.

Encouragement, support and wisdom of the latter would help build a strong and solid foundation, enabling the Light (Christ) in my life to continue to burn brightly, especially during darker times, which are inevitable. Life will always be unpredictable ... it's something all of us will experience during the course of our time here on earth. To possess consistent inner peace, it's critical to stay focused on the Light. John 3:21 says, *"But whoever lives by the truth comes into the light, so that it may be seen plainly **that what he has done has been done through God"*** (emphasis mine). This must be my predominant focus.

The first couple of years following the accident provided a base of knowledge, easing but not eliminating frustrations often swallowed up in unknowns. I was eager to explore the productive areas that would aid in my progression forward. I wasn't interested in a non-productive lifestyle that would rob me of God's abundant blessings, and Him the pleasure He found in creating this life of mine.

The optimistic decision to let my brain in its new capacity retrain me was going to require lifelong resolve. Adapting to each individual situation would continue to be a constant work in motion. I would need to assess many factors each and every day. I wanted and craved the Master's touch. I knew I needed His guidance and strength to be able to stand before Him one day, victorious in living abundantly the life He considered so precious. I do not want to stand before Him having wasted what He entrusted to my care. There will be no second chance to do it all over again.

I had previously enjoyed swimming, stroking out sixty laps every morning at our local recreation complex before work. Kip and our children worked out in the gym. A short while after the accident, I tried to go back to the pool, but the confusion of so much activity made it impossible to continue. Swimming in itself took so much concentration and coordination. With music and background talking, I quickly realized it wasn't even safe for me to continue.

The same type of situation occurred when I attempted to ride my bicycle. Yellow lines on the road, the noise and two-way direction of vehicles, plus sunshine spilling through the trees creating a kaleidoscope of shadows on the road, was far more than my brain could adequately process. The combination of stimuli overwhelmed me to the point of tears. Unsafe for me to continue, I got off my bike and walked the remaining distance to our daughter's home. My legs were weak as jelly, and I felt ready to pass out. After resting awhile, I found my strength returning, but Kip had to stop by her home after work to pick up my bicycle.

I knew I needed to find an alternative for exercise. I tried to go to a private gym, but again there was too much noise and excessive activity. I carried on in my search with an un-daunting determination that well defines my spirit at times. Several mornings I drove into town, combing out every fitness place I could think of. Becoming physically active again was pressing on me. I would stand outside the door and listen. Microphones, music, people shouting above the music, and the whirring of machines presented a real challenge to my quest. Without even one minute passing by, I knew beyond a shadow of a doubt I could not attend those places.

Another alternative had to be available. But what? Not wanting to leave any stone unturned, I thought through as many activities as I could, each one resulting in the same conclusion. The amount of commotion found in the visual and audible activity which takes place daily in our lives settles numbly into our awareness. Only through my newly acquired disability did I realize how busy and noisy our world has become!

I always enjoyed walking, so I endeavored to walk in our rural area. Again, the input of noise and the visual speed of cars and trucks made it dangerous for me. Extreme fatigue resulted from my inability to process it all adequately. I was somewhat frustrated and not all that impressed with how my brain was retraining me. All I was encountering were solid brick walls of defeat. With a hint of humour, I mused about how my brain was really re-*straining* me! After working outside in the orchard one day, I took a long, objective look around the one-and-a-half acre area. A new alternative presented itself. I was delighted by the possibilities. As my kids used to say, "It's a God thing!" I could make a walking path! Our property has been in my husband's family for decades. It had been cleared of overgrowth a few years earlier, and I was very familiar with it. Kip and I had just planted fruit trees, so it was still in the early stages of re-claiming true orchard status, yet it was perfect! Delight encompassed the core of my soul as I had at long last discovered an answer to my quest.

Great contentment washes over me as I delight in walking through this beautiful outdoor sanctuary. It is always available and it is free! For the most part, I can monitor my activity there. Always a good thing. Although repetitive, it is very safe and I now cover five kilometres every morning. I have experienced delightful satisfaction from having found a way to overcome this barrier. Another bonus? My weight is dropping and I feel healthier, both physically and emotionally, as the fresh air fills my lungs and clears out the cobwebs in my head, giving me a clearer focus. Do I feel "weird" when others see me walk circles and circles? I did in the beginning. But I had to evaluate whether it was worth the embarrassment of looking strange versus the benefit and victory I would experience over finding a way to clear this hurdle.

Often our perceptions of what others think are muddy. Every morning I have the opportunity to say good morning or send up a huge wave of my hand to the wonderful neighbours who pass by on their way to work or while they walk their own familiar route. I still have to monitor when it is best to walk, needing to avoid the buzzing of chainsaws, folks chopping wood, and other outdoor chores, but the very fact that a viable opportunity is available makes my heart soar with joy!

The closeness of my walking path makes it possible to be flexible with the times I walk. When one time doesn't work, it's right there waiting to be enjoyed at a more appropriate time.

Solutions are wonderfully encouraging, yet the discovery of solutions does not always guarantee further adjustments won't need to be made. My brain continues to retrain me, therefore fine-tuning is often required. I had obtained an exciting solution to my challenge. There was nothing that could possibly take me by surprise in this new discovery! Or was there?

One afternoon, I decided to go for my walk. Pressure-washing had been done on the driveway by a maintenance company in the morning, so I decided it was now quiet enough to walk. Even though I had remained inside while they worked for four hours, I was very tired, feeling drained by the continuous pulsating of the compressor. Stubbornly, I pushed aside the warning signals the specialist had cautioned about. I wanted some fresh air and needed some exercise. For some strange reason I decided to reverse my walking pattern so I wouldn't over-exercise one leg by continually walking in the same direction. I headed off to the right instead of the left. Within a minute or so, I found myself confused, recognizing the orchard but not really knowing where to walk next. My path was worn down, but I could not figure out how to stay on it. I kept wanting to turn off of it.

I ended up among some trees behind another building on the property, lost. I looked all around me, wondering how I was going to get out. I drew a deep breath and looked down, trying to mentally visualize the layout of our property. I worked very hard to remain calm, telling myself to think it all through carefully. Eventually, I ventured out from the trees and found my path again. Walking to the well-head a short distance away, I sat down, placing my head between my knees. I felt as though I would pass out and I didn't understand what had happened. Lack of awareness had engulfed me. I had no idea at the onset of my walk that the fatigue coupled with the change of direction would produce this end result!

There it was. One of the most applicable situations for discovering the immense importance of paying attention to the warning signs my brain was giving me. The constant pulsating noise of the compressor caused such fatigue I could not function in the simple activity of walking my route. I should have had a rest in complete peace and quiet before even attempting to tackle anything else. My brain had sent warning signals, but I deliberately chose to ignore them. It was a perfect example of how my brain needed to retrain me. I have not tried to walk the opposite way since. A friend of ours who lived on our property asked me why I didn't call for him. Honestly, I didn't have the energy or even the mindset to think of calling him. I was confused and I didn't know where to go until I saw the well-head.

Another example of irreverently ignoring the reality of my limitations came one summer not long ago. I had the wonderful inspiration to swim in the ocean in light of the fact I couldn't swim at the pool. I had great plans of purchasing a wetsuit to do "lengths" in the ocean early in the morning if the plan succeeded. I got really excited about this possibility, deciding a great fitness routine would evolve throughout the summer—swimming some mornings, walking other mornings. First I would test out the waters, so to speak.

The following morning, I slid into my bathing suit. I felt I had assessed the situation wisely and carefully. It was early, not busy on the beach yet, and the tide was out quite far. The waves seemed fairly minimal in size. Perfect for trying out my new idea! Due to my speed limitations, it took a while to actually get down to the ocean. I put on my sandals, grabbed my three-pound weights to use at the edge of the water, made sure I had my towel and the house key, then double and triple-checked that the door was locked. It had taken quite some time and energy just to get ready for this, so again I was somewhat worn down already. The waves had picked up and the surf had become quite boisterous.

I had always loved the motion of the waves. The direction of the waves indicated a southeasterly was blowing, and the water was always warmer then. Taking in the entire scene once I got down to the beach, I really knew full well that this was perhaps more than I should be attempting, especially alone. I felt unsettled with the sound of the surf and the rise and fall of the waves. It wasn't fear. It was a feeling of slight confusion, a feeling that was becoming an annoying companion at times.

Determination is a gift, stubbornness is a detriment. I once again made a bad choice, ignoring the warning signs that would have prevented the following from happening. I set my weights, towel and sandals aside and strode to the water. Wading to knee depth, I dove into the waves and swam three short lengths back and forth. By the third length, swimming away from the beach, I could tell something was very wrong. I stopped immediately. Rising out of the water, I attempted, unsuccessfully, to stand. My legs did not support me and I fell into the water. Fortunately I was not too deep and the slope of the beach was minimal. I tried to stand again but my legs prevented me from doing so. I felt dizzy, nauseous and somewhat scared as I crawled through the water, waves pushing me toward shore, thankfully. Arriving at the edge of the surf, I could do nothing but lay there. My legs would not move. I could not stand. I tried to sit up, but the nausea and dizziness persisted, so I remained lying down for a few more moments, waves beginning to break over my body.

Eventually I was able to sit for a few moments. Struggling to stand, I staggered over to my belongings. There were a couple of other people further down the beach, but I was safe and too embarrassed to ask for help. I rested a few more moments against the Big Rock, a family nickname for the particularly large boulder on the beach. Apprehensively, I wobbled up to our home. Opening the door with unsteady fingers, I put a towel around myself and lay down, tears flowing as my body trembled all over. What had happened out there?

Medical assessment concluded that my brain had gone into "overload." I had become quite tired just preparing for this venture. Mentally and physically. Vertigo had been a mild nuisance sometimes, so the elements of the situation likely triggered it also. The increased motion of the waves coupled with the breaking sound they made as they smashed on shore disoriented me. To top it off, I had been expecting my brain to relay synchronizing signals to my arms and legs so I could swim. Stimuli overload ensued. Too much activity was going in at one time and my brain couldn't sort it all out in proper sequence, throwing my entire body into turmoil.

Kip was *not* impressed with me. He was very concerned that a real tragedy could have taken place had the tide been going out instead of coming in. I knew I should have waited until he was home, but I was still seeking my independence and every time I looked out toward the beach it seemed the ocean was calling me out to play. I was already limited as to when I could go down on the beach, so the setting itself lured me toward the water. The result of what took place quickly convinced me to wait for Kip or someone else to be with me when I attempt to go down by the water from now on.

Sometimes the hard way, I have been harshly forced to acknowledge that yes, my brain is going to retrain me. Daily the door to several options is flung wide open. Decisions need to be made. I can choose to fight against the changes and warnings, putting myself at risk while also rousing frustration to the surface. These two vital lessons made me also realize what a selfish choice that would be, creating unfair concern in others. Another option would be to just give up trying, allowing life to pass by day after day. There was yet another choice. I could choose to accept the warning signals and adhere to them.

I knew what the Lord wanted. I also knew what my husband needed to avoid continual concern about me when he wasn't home. Learning to accept the retraining would require sensitivity and responsiveness to clearly defined signals, and it would hold a lot more promise for success than the ongoing disappointment and failure my stubbornness would keep hurling at me. Since that incident, I have done some more swimming in the ocean, when it's calm. I need help to cross over the millions of rocks and pebbles magnified beneath the water, the gentle current making them appear as though *they* are moving. Farther out, I am able to swim for a little while, always having someone close by. Still unsteady immediately afterward, I take time to sit on the logs for a bit until I feel able to walk sure-footedly again.

The same goes for kayaking or boating on the water. I need to get my land legs back before attempting to walk anywhere. I'm absolutely fine with the movement of the kayak on the water, but I need help when disembarking, taking time to sit and get my bearings before heading up to the house. It's not much different than what some folks experience when they are not used to movement on the water, the transition to walking on land again creating an unusual sensation.

However, these were activities I had participated in for years without any problem.

Following the accident, many of these previously familiar situations create such odd challenges. The challenges are not always critical. Some are just so unusual to experience, and I have to simply wait out the aftereffects, doing fine afterward. I had always loved to swim, jump and play in the ocean, particularly with my children. We would jump over each wave as it crashed into shore, our squeals barely heard above the pounding surf. There are many summer days when I see so many people doing exactly that, without any thought given to the enormous information highway inside their heads which processes every single audio and visual occurrence taking place around them. And, inside of them. How much we all take for granted until something changes within us, increasing our awareness of the intricacy of our human bodies.

I do remember at times what that freedom felt like, especially when I observe various scenarios. Sometimes I catch myself staring at such situations wishing I could return to those enjoyable activities as I had before, to once again be completely oblivious to the endless messages and signals that provide allowance for that "normal" activity. Yet it is only for a moment now that these feelings surface. I mentally move on, choosing not to lay waste the progress I *am* making.

I am fortunate to be able to figure out alternative ways to cope. I am still able to logically think through situations as long as I am given ample time to figure them out. Gratitude floods my soul for that remaining capability. I genuinely want to figure out as much as possible on my own using the gifts I still have. At the same time I want to openly receive new gifts God has waiting for me.

I've come to realize through the gift of time itself that it is imperative for me to accept, even embrace, the verity that the speed at which I process information is permanently damaged, forcing a much slower pace of message retrieval, resulting in a much slower pace of accomplishment. Grasping that truth and learning to be okay with it allows contentment with what I am able to accomplish, within the timeframe it is accomplished. Tapping into additional resources exposes fresh ideas and offers solid answers. My (re)training ground is expanding.

There is a constant need to be attentive to the signals designated by my brain. The progression is quite slow as I try to seek out alternatives for areas of definite deficiency. But, there is progression! The rewarding component of pacing myself and cooperating with the potential that remains is the increasing awareness of more frequent successes than failures. Assessing my capabilities and staying within my boundaries is crucial to moving forward with my life. I am eager to discover positive areas that will aid in my progression. Discarding doubts when they try to muddy the clarity of my focus requires constant skimming. I want to discover possibilities that await to grow me. I want to be grown.

Awareness delivers alternatives. Paying close attention to signs that relay messages, some of them painful, helps me understand more clearly those obvious areas I need to work on. Awareness of the blank look on my face during times of multiple conversations has challenged me to consciously work on softening my expression as others speak, even though I may not understand the discussion. Most who know me well speak one at a time so I can understand, but in gatherings where there are many people conversing I use my custom-designed ear plugs and remain close to Kip. He will often fill me in as the occasion arises. I am learning how to read the movement of people's lips when they speak to me directly, and when it is possible Kip and I will lead them over to a quieter corner where there is a higher possibility for me to join in the conversation.

My brain is retraining me, drawing me to a much better understanding of myself. It is crucial to seek out pertinent advice, and I work hard at finding ways to adapt to the effects of my injury. While this process is extremely challenging at times, yet also wonderfully rewarding, I am learning to pay close attention to the signals I receive from my brain. I am finally beginning to realize that identifying and staying within my boundaries allows me to be more refreshed and alert, increasing the quality of daily life. Frustration is not as common, although it can still be a thorn in my side. Retraining can seem endlessly time-consuming and my progress feels slow at times, or I may back-step a little. Accepting I will never be the same person I was before the accident has been extremely difficult, but through God's grace, His Word, and my own trial and error, I know I am heading in the right direction.

This new world I have entered is not one I would have chosen, but perhaps that is the most significant lesson here. My life is not my own. Rather, it has been designed by God the Father for His purpose. Isaiah 44:2 says, *"I am your Creator. You were in my care even before you were born"* (CEV). Redirecting my journey definitely caught my attention and has required me to fix my eyes on Him, practically moment by moment if I want to come through these changes victoriously. And I do want to be victorious.

The brain controls every aspect of our lives, sending signals and messages constantly. It is the motherboard of our human bodies, and it literally affects every part of our bodies. When it becomes permanently damaged, the degree of that damage determines what messages will be sent out, and when. Yet the brain is tucked away beneath the structure of our skull, so the damage itself is often masked. It cannot be touched, felt or visually seen, and sometimes that complicates situations and relationships tremendously. Certain limitations will forever be present; it has taken intense research, education and roaming through the darkness of ignorance to finally come to a healthy awareness of that truth.

I heavily depend on God for strength, courage, ideas and victory over my challenges. Being aware of my differences is sometimes scary, sometimes embarrassing and sometimes frustrating, but I am learning to perceive the differences as a uniqueness that allows my individuality. I am not always confident and I still often waver as new situations arise, but I am gradually accepting the process of learning how to let my brain retrain me as to what will work and what will not. I must continually surrender my self-will to try to change what cannot be changed. Seeking solutions daily prevents lethargy from robbing me of the abundant life God promises to give me. I must do my part with the abilities He has chosen to place within me.

I am still alive. I have a second chance on this earth to discover and access the power of the One Who created me, on a much deeper level. Furthermore, gratitude for what God is doing has begun to slip into my heart as I continue to progress with my eyes fixed on Jesus. To Him be the glory for His perfect design of each one of us. There is not one single life which has no worth.

PART FIVE

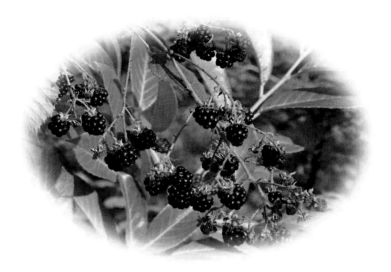

CREATED TO BEAR FRUIT

"You did not choose me, but I chose you
and appointed you to go and bear fruit—fruit that will last.
Then the Father will give you whatever you ask in my name."
(John 15:16)

1

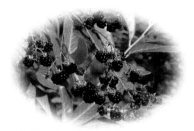

SPIRITUAL UNDERSTANDING

I AM ALIVE! GOD WAS NOT READY TO RECEIVE ME HOME YET. HIS ANGELS protected me from death that night—that I do know. The total write-off of my Plymouth Chrysler van and the way my driver's seat was twisted into two different directions attests to the miracle of God's protection. Some physical, muscular injuries did occur, and will continue to be an ongoing challenge, but it is the invisible brain injury which has drastically altered my life. From my perspective. But what about God's perspective? Did He alter His plan for my life midstream? Did He suddenly change His mind regarding the purpose He had chosen for me when He created me?

Psalm 139 has always been my favourite passage in the Bible. Psalm 139:16 says, *"All the days ordained for me were written in your book before one of them came to be." All* the days ordained for me! God had a purpose for my life before I was even born, that was clear and defined. He created me and the original plan He started with has not changed.

God is changeless. He is one-hundred percent trustworthy and He is absolutely faithful.

As far back as I can remember, I have always loved the Lord. I have trusted Him and I have witnessed His enduring faithfulness countless times throughout my life. The injuries resulting from this accident unquestionably turned my world upside-down, but has it made any difference in God's purpose for my life? Did He erase and replace my life's purpose halfway through my life's activity log? Not according to His Word in Psalm 139.

I am just beginning to understand and appreciate the vastness of God's power. He is constant, never changing. As I pursue spiritual understanding, this reveals to me that my accident did not come as a shock or surprise to God so that panic-stricken, He magically prevented my death because it would mess things up for Him. First of all, God doesn't panic and He is never under pressure. This is of enormous comfort to me when life dishes out some pretty hefty blows and I wonder how I am ever going to cope. Confidently trusting that life cannot dole out any surprises for the One Who created and cares for me blankets my heart with a peace that is beyond human understanding.

Almighty God, my Heavenly Father, knew every breath and step of life I was going to take before I was even born! Psalm 139:16 says, *"Like an open book, you watched me grow from conception to birth; all the stages of my life were spread out before you, The days of my life all prepared before I'd even lived one day"* (The Message). God the Creator miraculously sculpted and moulded my life. His desire was for me to simply be, His purpose antedated before He breathed life into me. That truth validates my worthiness, saturating my whole being with excitement!

The accident and difficulties arising from it force me to depend on *Him* instead of myself. I am here for His purpose, not my own and I am truly grateful He is in control of my life. What a mess things would be if I were the one in complete control! Only Almighty God has the supernatural power to be in ultimate and complete control of all life, mine included.

One particularly rough time, when this "intruder" was still nameless, God used my husband to teach both of us a very crucial lesson. Preparing dinner, I placed chicken wings onto a baking sheet. A serious situation had recently taken place and tears would not hold back even though I told them to. The salty floodgates burst wide open. Difficult questions had been asked, for which I had no answers. I did not know how to move past this particularly large stumbling block. The pain in my soul would not subside and I did not know what to do, or how to change it.

Kip picked up the baking sheet that was covered in little chicken wings. He pushed it toward me and said, "Take it, Kathie." I raised my eyes to meet his, questioning why he wanted me to put this baking sheet in the oven, right now! Dinner could wait! He pushed it toward me again and said, "Kath, this is like the situation at hand. Everything feels broken and jumbled into a million pieces, just like this bunch of chicken wings. Disjointed. So, take the chicken plate, Kathie."

I resisted him. "Why?" I asked. He sternly told me again to take the baking sheet from him and when I did we both were sobbing.

He said to me, *"That* is what we do with this situation and every other situation that seems way beyond our understanding or capabilities. We surrender it to the Lord. He removes the shattered broken pieces from our hearts and replaces them with His peace. We need to trust Him and fully surrender what we cannot manage, asking Him to bring understanding to our hearts. In *His* time."

I pray I will never forget that incredible lesson as long as I live! Satan still tries to rattle our world with bouts of confusion, doubt and "whispers" of not measuring up, but since that day we determinedly "give the chicken plate" to our Lord God Almighty. In Him there is only peace and order. There is hope of total restoration for the soul willing to surrender chaos, uncertainty or "broken pieces" to His loving care. It's crucial to be proactive, doing everything we can do at that time. But there are and always will be circumstances in which we need to lift up to Him what is beyond our human capabilities. External chaos, uncertainty, and jumbled pieces may remain, but God will navigate our hearts to a safe and restful harbour of spiritual peace.

Each person has unique, individual gifts from God, and learning to cultivate those gifts brings glory to Him. I am beginning to realize how busy this world is and how much simpler and quieter my world has become. Through this season of change, I am understanding how important it is to comfortably embrace alone time with God, to earnestly seek Him, to listen to His voice. Realistically, we cannot hear God speaking to us when our lives are in high-gear from the instant we wake up in the morning until we close our eyes in exhaustion at night. Where then does God fit in? Is it spiritually healthy to *fit* Him in? How do we grab even a moment with Him while reeling on the rollercoaster of life? Do we even breathe His name with love? Do we even breathe His name?

Time alone with God brings peace, security, answers, understanding and true fullness of life. I am gaining a stronger sense of security as I begin to understand that I don't *need* to be surrounded by others to truly know who I am. Psalm 46:10 says, *"Be **still**, and know that I am God"* (emphasis mine). I am learning to understand the powerful significance of being still, of setting time aside for my Lord. It is the only way to understand His purpose for my life. It is the only way to truly know Him.

I cannot intimately know someone if I don't set aside time with them. They cannot intimately know me if we don't take time to share together. There is tremendous security in the trust built between loyal friends who schedule time for each other. By the same token I cannot know God if I don't spend time in His Holy Word listening for Him to speak as I wait in silence and expectation. Our relationship cannot be bonded tightly if I refrain from sharing my intimate self with Him. These times of vulnerability hold tremendous power and strength. Unlike human insolence toward vulnerability, God treasures my openness and uses our time together to grow me, not just on the surface but deep within the core of who I am. Having this security and peace feels refreshing. I am comfortable being alone with God and I am becoming comfortable being alone with me. Looking in the mirror, I am no longer baffled by who I see in the reflection. I do not see a stranger anymore, and I am becoming at ease with the woman smiling back at me.

While preaching recently, a dear friend of ours gave a beautiful illustration of what I now experience, only he took it a little farther. He encouraged us as believers to envision the Lord standing right behind us when we stop to really look at ourselves in the mirror. This illustration opened my eyes to an even bigger awareness. Being alone does not signify loneliness. I am never truly alone, because Christ is always with me. The Lord has promised to be my "rear guard" at all times. Isaiah 58:8–9 declares, *"Then your light will break forth like the dawn, and your healing will quickly appear; then your righteousness will go before you, and the glory of the LORD will be your rear guard. Then you will call, and the LORD will answer; you will cry for help, and he will say: Here am I."* I have called on Him, many times. He is my rear guard, and He has always been faithful.

This journey is not just about me; other lives interweave with mine. The quest for personal growth is essential for progress to take place, but an unhealthy self-focus must not enter into the equation. Self-focus is a wasteful trait and in itself does lead to loneliness. I have pondered how I can share Christ and all that He is when I have so many limitations. Limitations which rigidly limit social interaction with others. Once again the answers come in the form of taking the focus off myself and my circumstances. I need to ask myself, "What does God want me to learn so I can share Him with others?" James 1:2–3 says, *"Consider it a sheer gift, friends, when tests and challenges come at you from all sides. You know that under pressure, your faith-life is forced into the open and shows its true colors"* (The Message). I've clearly been aware of the importance of how I handle what has happened in my life, since it reveals to everyone around me just how real and deep my faith is. This is a huge responsibility, since I proclaim Jesus Christ as Lord of my life.

In the early stages of my brain injury, I handled this responsibility very poorly. First of all, I didn't understand what was happening to me. Secondly, I succumbed to a common misconception as to what it means to be a committed Christian. If I was *truly* walking with the Lord, I should have been able to overcome anything, shouldn't I? Particularly something which seemed to be "all in my head." I tried so hard to evict the stranger causing havoc in my life, yet was failing miserably. Blundering through each day, I tried to convince others (and myself) that God would give me strength to overcome the effects of the accident.

Realistically I nearly passed out at times, tears flowed when I couldn't understand or execute the simplest matters, and frustration mounted because I continued to remain an unwilling participant in a world that was foreign to me. I couldn't change what was happening. I couldn't will my previous way of living back, and I was very aware that there was some reproach toward the way I was responding to certain situations. How could Christ possibly be honoured in a life that had become filled with such chaos? It was a very difficult time and I had begun to heavily doubt the depth of my proclaimed faith.

I realize now that it has taken several years for God to refine my understanding. I knew something was terribly wrong following the accident, yet I didn't know what. I had done a lot of talking *to* the Lord, but had not done a whole lot of listening. There were expectations for me to resume life as it had been prior to the accident. I would collapse with utter exhaustion trying to meet those unrealistic expectations. Aching inside, I felt I was letting God down enormously by not being able to do the things I used to. How could I ever reflect God's faithfulness when I was unable to function in "normal" activities and gatherings? How could I ever be used by God again? How would others ever see the magnificence of Who He is when my life, a believer's life, remained seemingly untouched by His healing hand?

I believe God chose not to intervene during that time of internal turmoil. He allowed me to bounce around in that emotional maze of instability and self-doubt, yet He remained right by my side. Had I reached for His hand, I would have found it already outstretched. Due to my injuries I was not able to reclaim what had been lost in the accident. Yet I was trying to, through my own efforts. I falsely believed the only way I could prove God's faithfulness to others was through a miraculous return to the old me. God knew otherwise. He knew His purpose for my life, and returning to my former lifestyle, as great as I thought it was, was not in His plan.

My spiritual vision became extremely blurred. My attempts to do what could no longer be done were leading me down a destructive path. Heedless of the permanence of my injury, my morning thoughts would be geared to overcoming this "glitch" in my life. God knew my personal combat and He knew the outcome, thus His allowance of the internal battle raging inside of me. I needed to be completely broken before Him in order for Him to start putting the pieces together again. When that time came, the canvas of my heart was wiped pure and clean. Only then could He inaugurate His purpose for this part of my journey.

Life is not what society makes it out to be; it is what God creates it to be. I am beginning to finally grasp what that means. Serving others is serving Christ, fulfilling His purpose even if it is serving one person at a time. As Christians we can tend to be zealous about winning hundreds of folks to Christ. Successfully serving Christ is not determined by how busy we are, how many people we entertain at one time, how many functions we attend, or how much money we give to charities or His Church. What does matter to Him is how we serve others in His name, according to His leading, despite our limitations.

Billy and Ruth Bell Graham's daughter Anne Graham Lotz said this about her parents: "My father preaches sermons to the masses, reaching thousands; my mother talks to individuals, loving them one by one."[2] I often think of her reflective words. Her mother passionately shared the gospel, touching individual lives, loving them one by one. Anne's reflection ignited a spark in me. God has a specific calling for each one of us. Recognizing my limitations as special gifts from God is what He expects from me. Using those gifts is what brings honour to Him.

Satan tries to whisper lies to me, attempting to change my focus from God's purpose to his destructive initiatives. Under the dark cloak of falsehood, he suggests to me that I am a failure because I am unable to live life in the capacity I used to. He readily appears during vulnerable times, eager to convince me that I am letting God and others down. He must be stopped. The only truth worth focusing on is that God knows my heart. I try with all of my soul to be who God wants me to be and to do what He asks of me to do. I must cover myself every morning with God's armour. Ephesians 6:10–11 emphasizes, *Finally, be strong in the*

---

[2] Anne Graham Lotz (with permission), Decision Magazine, Billy Graham Evangelistic Association, Special Commemorative Issue 2007

Lord and in his mighty power. Put on the full armor of God so that you can take your stand against the devil's schemes."

Once again I look to Paul as he pleads with God in 2 Corinthians to remove what was ailing him. With personal interest, it intrigues me that God chose to allow the ailment to remain with Paul. He also used it to work through Paul. Paul had been a very self-sufficient man, and I can relate to his distress in some ways. I had also been very independent, now at times I am very dependent. I am fascinated with the way God speaks to Paul in 2 Corinthians 12:9, *"But he said to me, 'My grace is sufficient for you, for my power is made perfect in weakness.'"* Paul was constantly reminded of his need for God's power and strength because his own physical body was letting him down. Notwithstanding some personal turmoil, Paul remained a willing servant, surrendering his pride and will to be moulded and used by God, ailment and all. It was Paul's goal and deep desire to know how to live and become like Christ Jesus. He genuinely desired to be who God wanted him to be.

Despite all that had transpired in his life, Paul had received total cleansing through the blood of Jesus Christ. Starting fresh, he says in Philippians 3:13–14, *"But one thing I do: Forgetting what is behind and straining toward what is ahead, I press on toward the goal to win the prize for which God has called me heavenward in Christ Jesus."* Christian living requires a commitment to Christ with a vision to honour Him in character and integrity. A vision to be *used* by Almighty God. Through this vision we can sort out what is truly real in our lives, and where authentic worth really resides. Paul stresses something crucial at the beginning of his statement, *"But one thing I do: Forgetting what is behind and straining toward what is ahead..."* I believe Paul was refusing to look behind at the areas of failure in his life. He knew how important it was to fix (position) his eyes on Jesus Christ, the Author and Perfecter of his faith. It was the only way God could truly use him.

As aforementioned, I am realizing that limitations are only what I perceive them to be. The disability is there, and the newly acquired limitations are present, but would I view these changes as limitations had I always lived with them? Or would I have learned to adapt to them naturally? This understanding is critical to moving forward in the journey God has planned for me. It is a much different path than I was coasting on prior to my car accident. Yet the sharp turn in the pathway was the direction God wanted me to travel. The accident did not throw God a curveball. He was absolutely in control of every single thing that took place that night.

I marvel at the direction this path is taking me. At times it seems less comfortable and the growing pains are not always easy to accept, but I am gaining an awesome understanding of what it means to completely surrender my life to God. To completely trust Him. Open before me are avenues of opportunity leading in a different direction than I would have otherwise taken. I would never have been aware of the many things shaping my life now as a result of my disability. Stronger spiritual awareness is leading to glorification of God as I embrace His unwavering faithfulness! Everything that happens to us in life has been authorized by God, even when we don't understand by way of human understanding.

I cherish the fact that God's Holy Spirit is still working in me. I accepted Christ as my Saviour when I was very young. At that time I became a new creation, a brand new person. The old me no longer remained. I was given new life through Christ Jesus. The powerful truth of that decision hasn't changed. I am still Kathie, the woman who loves Jesus with all of her heart. I always will be. God's Holy Spirit is alive and very active in my life. That doesn't guarantee earthly freedom from difficulties, sin and struggles, but it does guarantee spiritual freedom upon repentance.

God is supreme and powerful! His strength is revealed through my weaknesses. Only by experiencing weaknesses can I ever truly understand the sufferings of another. Only then can I have full and genuine compassion for another who may be struggling without divine hope, wondering what his or her worth measures up to anymore. With God there is no measuring stick to calculate our worth. We are worthy simply because we are His children.

As the years progress, God has been shedding light on two kinds of understanding for me. Human understanding and spiritual understanding. My human understanding has been based on knowledge, education, awareness, insight and perception. Even more beneficial has been the discovery of spiritual understanding. This offers a bounty of possibilities which far surpasses human understanding. The awareness and focus are different, as God reveals many truths through eyes that are fixed on Him.

Spiritual understanding swings doors of opportunity wide open to serve others no matter how small or large the human capability is. When God calls us to service, He will provide everything needed. Our human understanding may cast doubt on our effectiveness for God, but it is then that spiritual understanding embraces the promise of what God can and will do through us. It is up to us to always have *"Ears that hear and eyes that see"* (Proverbs 20:12). Tuning in to God and His will provides understanding on a most magnificent and spiritual level.

2

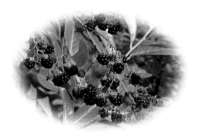

Changing Focus

When adversity changes our world it is imperative to go before Christ to reevaluate our journey. Growing in my spiritual walk with God, I have become much more aware of the dangers that lie in focusing on myself and the difficulties of my circumstances. This inward way of thinking seriously limits my appreciation and acknowledgement of the wonderful things He is doing in my life. It places restrictions on His freedom to use me for His purpose. Engrossed in personally overcoming the challenges, I do not open myself freely to Him. Proverbs 21:30 says, *"There is no wisdom, no insight, no plan that can succeed against the LORD."* A change of focus, looking upward instead of inward, is a healthy beginning.

Many loved ones and friends have accepted and embraced the permanent changes in my life. Because of their love, support, and encouragement I am moving forward with confidence. By God's grace, my intelligence and ability to reason remains intact. Gratitude flows from my heart as the characteristics of love, humour, faith, faithfulness and trustworthiness continue to be active in my personality. Building others up through sincere words and deeds of encouragement often has a boomerang effect, bestowing a personal gift often not recognized. It is the gift of contentment. Yes, indeed, life retains immense value when lived in service toward others.

A brand new chapter has been unfolding. God has new work for me to do. It is my responsibility to listen very carefully to His voice and to follow His leading. This can only be accomplished in a heart that is willing. Romans 12:1–2 says,

> *Therefore, I urge you, brothers, in view of God's mercy, to offer your bodies as living sacrifices, holy and pleasing to God—this is your spiritual act of worship. Do not conform any longer to the pattern of this world, but be transformed by the renewing of your mind. Then you will be able to test and approve what God's will is—his good, pleasing and perfect will.*

Initially, this new chapter required a thorough and lengthy self-evaluation of exactly where I was standing before God. I needed to assess all the qualities that remained fertile in my life, and it was extremely important to seek pertinent advice from others. Words of encouragement and wisdom made a significant difference in my resolve to progress confidently. I refer to Proverbs 15:22 often: *"Plans fail for lack of counsel, but with many advisers they succeed."*

This evaluation process began approximately three years after the accident. The first step, and one of the hardest, was to contact a psychologist/counsellor who was familiar with brain injuries and their effects. My physician had given me her name and phone number. I carried it around with me for quite a while, wanting to call but afraid to call. I had to get past the notion that if I truly loved the Lord I wouldn't need to see a psychologist. I had begun to realize, however, that I needed a private place to talk where I could honestly reveal my struggles without being criticized or judged. The phone felt like a lead pipe in my hand when I finally made the decision to call her.

This wonderful counsellor was the first of a few whom God led me to. Through detailed and open discussions with her I gained valuable insight about my disability, my strengths and my focus. It was extremely freeing to sit with someone who really knew many of the struggles I was battling as a result of this disability. She counselled others experiencing similar difficulties, and it was comforting to talk with someone who understood what I was trying to explain. Knowledge of my struggles and affirmation of my adaptations increased my confidence, and I was tremendously encouraged by the professional information I received. That first unsettling step was instrumental in enabling me to move forward with much more confidence.

Talking openly with a professional who knew the effects of my disability, and understood them, greatly eased my frustrations. Tapping into other credible professionals who were familiar with the challenges I was experiencing lifted an enormous load off my shoulders. There were tangible situations to address and I didn't have to try to figure them out on my own! My brain injury wasn't the only one that existed, although it felt like it when I tried to fit into a normal situation. Various professionals were conversant with the roadblocks and were readily accessible when I faced one head-on. For me, the roadblocks were brand new, but the experts were familiar with them. They identified the unknowns I was experiencing, and together we worked through many of them.

I am so thankful God gave me the guidance and courage to pick up that phone to call the first counsellor. God's leading brought me to someone who was positive, knowledgeable and extremely encouraging. During our sessions it was evident I was progressing extremely well. Those willing to accept this disability and the permanent changes it brought recognized the progress. Myself included. I had been making a real effort to progress and finally those efforts were acknowledged and applauded. It was a strong affirmation that life could only get better.

The next step was to recognize my disability as an opportunity to help others. A major stumbling block had been my inability to foresee my life weaving amongst others' lives. I had been looking at this obstacle from an unrealistic angle. Without professional guidance, counsel or proper understanding of my limitations, I had been trying to find a solution to the unsolvable. An ongoing concern was my inability to socialize in group settings, in the manner I had before. However, when I discussed this with pertinent sources, I was introduced to the optimistic plausibility of interacting with folks one on one. Another new door opened and this consideration certainly was worth investigating and experimenting with! A glimmer of light started to shine on the pathway of possibilities.

This is where pure excitement flows through my veins. The process has been lengthy and will continue to evolve for a lifetime. But there are finally strands of light shining on a million tomorrows! Coming to terms with what has happened, and all that the climb has entailed to this point, is producing change in my life. Positive change. I could never have envisioned where this journey would lead while engulfed in the swamp of confusion and turmoil immediately following the accident. Yet in order to be renewed and refined it was crucial for me to go through that process. Physical changes took place during the accident and a period of adjustment was necessary to gain understanding and acceptance of those changes.

I am gradually becoming comfortable with who I am now, learning to accept and even embrace the changes. Coupled with that mindset is the intense desire to seek out really neat ways to adapt to various situations. If ever there was opportunity for brain-testing, this is it! It requires focused cognitive thinking to find solid solutions to many daily challenges. There are times when I soar like a bird, with interaction and solutions producing positive results. One example is our motor home—a familiar and disability-friendly retreat while travelling. Highway driving produces a hodgepodge of activity, so I wear an eye-mask when my brain pleads for a rest. Unable to dine in restaurants, we prepare our own meals, always packing a candle for ambiance at dinnertime. Million-dollar views enrich the dining experience. Kip and I enjoy meeting fellow travellers, yet I am able to recharge my energy batteries at any time. Each fall, we travel to Alberta, and because of our private little kitchen, I am able to contribute to shared mealtimes at my aunt's home. Jet-setting travel is unfeasible, however our decision to invest in a motor home has empowered us to reclaim our favourite pastime: adventure.

There are also times when limitations curtail my efforts, and alternatives evade discovery. My mother broke her femur at the age of eighty-five. The situation was critical. Following surgery, she developed a blood clot and had to remain in the emergency ward of an Alberta hospital. The intensity of those surroundings would have magnified the effects of my disability, so I was not able to be with her. My heart ached with guilt, my mind swirled endlessly to find ways to help her despite the distance, and my arms longed to comfort her. I felt powerless during such a traumatic event.

This situation callously exposed the impediment of my disability in an area that had never been challenged so profoundly. I had to accept there were no feasible solutions to this heart-wrenching test. Had there been, I know God would have opened my eyes to them. Surrendering all, I placed my precious mother into His loving care.

Yet discouragement doesn't surface as quickly anymore. Challenges become viewed as beneficial instead of disparaging, and optimism seeks out workable solutions.

Boundaries are becoming more healthy and manageable as I figure out how far I can push myself and where I need to set limits. Most important is the discipline to *keep* within those boundaries, admittedly an area of constant struggle and evaluation. The price I pay when crossing those boundaries is high, and I am reminded of that the hard way. Reality can be life's greatest teacher and I am learning to become a very attentive student!

Hungry for God's Word, I begin my day communing with Him. I'm trying to pay special attention to the bounty of His magnificent blessings. His perfect scheduling. His incredible faithfulness. In the quiet of the morning, alone in the presence of Almighty God, peace floods my soul. I feel strong to start the day and I feel joy and anticipation for what awaits. Perhaps nothing particularly special will take place. Yet if I truly look for God throughout the day, whatever that day holds, I will find Him there in even the smallest detail. It matters not whether the day is gratifying or taxing. He remains by my side through it all. He is my constant companion, my dearest friend. He is also Lord of my life and I trust Him completely. There is a deep longing in my heart to share these truths with others. Becoming more secure in who I am, coming to terms (for the most part) with the swirling whirlwind of unwanted change in my life, I crave to share God's power, love and faithfulness with others.

Through this journey, I am just beginning to recognize God's leading toward a certain calling. It is one I would not have had time for prior to the switch in the track. My life before the accident was wonderful, and I thank God for the enormous blessings that washed over every aspect of it, particularly with my family. The first change of focus was unsettling and unwanted as it intruded callously at the time of the accident. Not by choice it was internal and inward due to an instantaneous lack of ability to function as I had just the day before, just moments before.

The subsequent three years demanded intense concentration toward self-discovery. I had to figure out how to adapt to changes that were permanent and through God's grace I gradually began to accept this new way of life. An internal focus was necessary in order to understand the disability and how to proactively work *with* it. Along the way, I grew to be a willing servant toward His refining. More recent years have sprouted a new focus. A really healthy, outward focus. This is what God was preparing me for during the earlier years. It was very painful, but God brought me through it. Even better, He brought me through it victoriously. I am experiencing tremendous joy as He opens doors and windows and everything else, allowing me to focus on and serve others in His name.

Changing focus from the upheaval of my circumstances to compassion for another's anguish deepens my sensitivity and conveys genuine and sincere understanding. My concern for others has always been authentic, but truly understanding their feelings or pain on the same level was impossible. I couldn't fully comprehend the heartaches of others until I underwent my own journey of questions, turmoil, heartache and pain.

Peter speaks of the importance of using our God-given gifts to help others see Christ. Nowhere does the Bible say, "Only if you have this or that ability can you be used by God." 1 Peter 4:10 says, *"Each one should use **whatever gift** he has received to **serve others,** faithfully administering God's grace in its various forms"* (emphasis mine). God's grace comes through various forms; however, rarely, if ever does it come in the form of a life untouched by heartache.

Christ stressed servanthood throughout His ministry. He is the Son of God and His "title" far surpasses any human title worthy of recognition. Yet Christ our Lord personally displayed how to serve God daily. Joining together with companions to share a meal, He removed his outer clothing, wrapped a towel around his waist, then knelt down to wash His disciples' feet. Can you imagine the dirt, dust (and other undesirable grime) on their feet after travelling along dusty and rugged roads all day? Roads which animals also used? Can you grasp the confusion in His disciples' hearts when their Lord stooped to do a servant's job? The same Lord Who healed the sick and blind, performing miracle upon miracle?

God's Holy Word describes this humble act and its meaning in John 13:12–17:

When he had finished washing their feet, he put on his clothes and returned to his place. "Do you understand what I have done for you?" he asked them. "You call me 'Teacher' and 'Lord,' and rightly so, for that is what I am. Now that I, your Lord and Teacher, have washed your feet, you also should wash one another's feet. I have set you an example that you should do as I have done for you. I tell you the truth, no servant is greater than his master, nor is a messenger greater than the one who sent him. Now that you know these things, you will be blessed if you do them.

How I want to be blessed! Yet, even more so I want *to* bless—others! And, I can. Opportunities abound every single day to serve someone else or to lift another's heart.

The largest treasure chest of blessings comes directly from the heart of one who shows humility and compassion in their expression of servanthood. This is not a symbol of weakness. Humility is a symbol of inner strength. It expresses confidence in Whom I am ultimately serving, Jesus Christ. It does not grow in a heart intent on gaining "points" through the administration of good deeds. That would be a self-centered motive. Servanthood in the truest sense comes from a willing heart whose sole purpose is to glorify Christ in tangible ways.

Servanthood reflects the love of God. It says to another, "You are more important than I." That's not stating a lack of self-worth. On the contrary. Uplifting another through words or acts of kindness silently affirms that I am comfortable with who I am, in Christ. I don't have to be first. I don't have to prove how good I am. I don't have to boast about the "wonderful" things I have done. I discover ultimate spiritual security in Christ when I finally embrace the attitude that life is not all about me. Jesus said in the above passage, *"You call me 'Teacher' and 'Lord,' and rightly so, for that is what I am."* Christ's knowledge of Who He was opened the door freely to confidently serve others without any status barrier.

Throughout Scripture we are called to serve. To be servants. To represent God through ordinary acts of kindness. The list of possibilities is endless. Unearthing creative ways to encourage another can also produce personal joy, without a personal motive. There is nothing sweeter in this whole world than to see a smile take shape on a face that was full of anguish and pain, to hear laughter as it replaces heart-wrenching sobs. For the most part we can't change the situation, but Christ can always use us to lighten a spirit, draw out a smile, ease an emotional load, or display kindness to a complete stranger expecting nothing, absolutely nothing, from them in return. There may also be times when Christ calls us to weep with others as they weep, to be a companion in their pain. Opportunities to serve Him may sometimes require no words but rather shared tears, hugs and a time to be silent. A time to just listen.

Regardless of our capabilities or *lack* of certain capabilities, God can and will use us. Remembering who I am in Christ enables me to kneel before another in service. With humility. My ultimate goal is to bring glory to my Lord through an unfolded, unselfish focus toward someone else. God is working on changing my focus. Looking upward with the deep desire to serve others beats looking inward at my own deficits, hands-down. I am a willing student who is eager to learn and I am grateful to Christ my Lord for remaining the ever-patient teacher.

May I always remain worthy to be His humble servant.

"He must become greater; I must become less." (John 3:30)

3

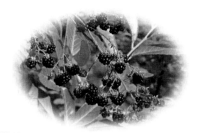

Developing Character

I HAVE ALWAYS WANTED GOD THE FATHER TO BE THE CENTRE OF MY LIFE. I have not always succeeded in making Him a priority, but I have tried to remain faithful to His Word, aware of His Presence. He is Omnipotent, all-seeing and all-knowing. I could hide nothing from Him. I was never afraid of that truth, perhaps being too comfortable at times, deliberately choosing to sin against Him.

Like most of us, I had personal dreams and goals, which is a healthy way to live. But when they exclude God's plans, even by way of innocence or ignorance, they become entirely self-focused. I had always enjoyed sharing what God was doing in my life, but it wasn't until this accident that I truly experienced the very essence of His Presence and faithfulness. He has been opening my spiritual eyes to the extremely personal relationship readily available through Jesus.

Seeking contentment through avenues excluding a desire for God's involvement can foster a false sense of self-made success and security. We may or may not pray. If we do pray, we may feign a quest for His guidance yet surreptitiously mutter, "I am handling everything fine thanks, Lord. Please don't rattle my world too drastically. I've got a comfortable hold on it just as it is."

When our self-righteous life begins to crumble, and it will crumble at some point, bitterness encroaches because we can no longer control the things around us. Arriving at that junction, we finally concede that we need our Lord and Saviour to truly live abundant lives. Some folks never do gain insight to the reality that only Christ can make us truly whole. Without Him, battles of the human will jeopardize God's gift of abundant life, putting relationships and, sometimes, lives at risk.

Claiming to be self-made only leads to the highway of self-destruction. We are expected to be proactive in our walk with Him, making the most of our abilities and strengths. He wants us to give our best and He wants us to experience success. But ultimately, only our Living God can bring us safely through trials and situations beyond our humanness. Only when we acknowledge the need to completely surrender our very lives to Him do the tumultuous seas of helplessness seem to lose their overpowering strength.

If the seas of life were always calm, I may attempt to steer my ship without God's help. Cautiously, I would try to maneuver it, hoping to avoid rough seas of challenge, vulnerability and perhaps heartache. However, such avoidance could falsely produce a sense of self-made success. I would miss endless opportunities for growth, and God's uniquely designed purpose for my life would be hopelessly lost. I would never experience the power of God's intervention and majesty. I would miss out on witnessing endless miracles and the likelihood for total destruction from a demolishing wave of distress would be high.

Life free of challenges and trials will not produce character. When those waves of frustration, loneliness, sadness, powerlessness and concern crash over me, only God can pull me up and direct me to safe, calm waters again. Psalm 29:11 says, *"The LORD gives strength to his people; the LORD blesses his people with peace."* Peace is that safe shore our souls arrive on after battling a violent storm which threatened to destroy us. There is a sense of calm. There is a sense of absolute trust, and there is the realization that God truly is in control.

God is developing my character, making me a much stronger woman. He is helping me feel, really feel, deep concern for others and how to reach out beyond my own world. So many people are hurting or struggling right in our midst. The question, "How are you?" is shallow if there is no desire to hear any response other than "Fine." So wrapped up in our own complexities, we do not even recognize pain in another's life. If we do recognize it, we shy away, not wanting that "negativity" to taint the joy of our lives.

Harsh lessons learned throughout the preceding years brought me renewed awareness and sensitivity. Prior to the accident, I believe I was also guilty of the above-mentioned oversights at times. I was so grateful for the blessings in my life that perhaps I was wearing invisible blinders, blinders that may have blocked out the pain swirling around in another's life. I've had to ask forgiveness from the Lord for that inward focus, which likely prevented me from outwardly recognizing someone else's hurts.

This revelation made me realize that I only partially understood what God asks of us. I have always delighted in making someone else feel really special without others knowing I've done something, sometimes without that person even knowing I was involved. I absolutely love the verse in Matthew 6:3–4 that says, *"Do not let your left hand know what your right hand is doing, so that your giving may be in secret. Then, your Father, who sees what is done in secret, will reward you."* I know Jesus promises a reward from God in this passage, and it is a wonderful promise given to an obedient heart. But it is not personal recognition or the promise of a reward that is the key to this passage; it is really the reference to serving others.

In my view, the most exciting message held within that passage is the joy of doing something wonderful for someone else without anyone knowing about it! Society thrives on receiving recognition for helping others. Particularly at Christmas. The flood gates of generosity open wide as folks can't do enough to help those "less fortunate." Contemplating that for a moment, how do we know about the details of those gifts? Tremendous publicity, that's how! Recognition is not wrong. Help provided to so many people is astounding, and recipients are tremendously grateful. In some cases the generosity challenges others to do the same. When good things are done there is reason to celebrate! What I believe Jesus is saying, however, is that we please God enormously when giving to others in secret or without proclamation. It is a sign of humility. There is no personal desire or motivation for praise. What is done quietly (in secret) offers no platform for self-elevation or misguided competitiveness. The only motive is to bring joy or much-needed help to another human being. The motive is pure.

Beyond tangible and monetary gift-giving lies something even more valuable. It is the jewel of trustworthiness. When someone feels secure enough to confide in us, we must have wide-open ears and a tightly closed mouth. God calls us to honour Him, and one of the most compelling ways to do that is to become a trusted confidant. Making this area a priority in your life not only cultivates deep and lasting relationships, it also develops integrity and character on your part.

Trustworthiness and protection of confidences reveals the depth of your walk with God. It is impossible to walk with the Father of Light, Almighty God, while cementing one foot in the dark with the father of lies, Satan. Numerous Scriptures reference the correlation between character, integrity and truth. One Scripture verse is particularly relevant: Proverbs 11:13 says, *"A gossip betrays a confidence, but a trustworthy man keeps a secret."* God's instructions are very clear.

I am grateful He still calls me to serve others. Blundering through a seemingly endless sea of trials and difficulties has roused opportunities for service which are somewhat distinctive because of my disability. I have a deeper understanding of gyrating emotions which can result after a life-changing event occurs, whatever it may be. Until I experienced them personally, I did not know how to relate. Taking each new step, I often ask my Father to remove the one-sided mirror of self-focus. This dramatically changes my perspective and enables me to "be there" with ears that hear, eyes that see, and a heart that safeguards confidences.

My life's journey has embarked on some rough and rocky roads. It hasn't been heartbreak-free or trouble-free. Kip and I encountered difficulties and trials in our lives, individually as well as together, but never had we experienced total chaos such as spun our lives around so feverishly the past few years. Only by going through the process described in previous chapters have we been able to get a handle on what God is doing in us and through us. There are folks who have suffered much greater tragedies than I have, and I don't want to ever minimize the enormity of their struggles. It has taken all this time to come to terms with my own brain injury, let alone a disability much more profound, or a loss more profound. But I am seeing and understanding how God is using this disability, my disability, to bring me to a much deeper place of compassion. I can now identify with the fear, helplessness and grief which occur during a loss, of any kind.

Allowed unbarred access, God continues to grow and strengthen my character. This complete openness to Him discloses my need for Him. I willingly said, "Yes" to being remoulded. Never say "Yes" lightly to God. Be prepared for some action! When you say "Yes," consenting to something as profound as being remoulded by the very One Who holds your life in His hands, you better hold on tight! Growing can be very uncomfortable, even painful at times.

God has given me freedom to choose. Yet, what a tragedy if I resented or resisted His refining touch. What enormous loss if it were ever refused. My growth would be severely stunted, and God's exciting plan for my life would be tragically thwarted because of my foolish stubbornness and fear of what He might really require of me. That choice would produce a very empty and lonely life. Thank God He waited patiently for my heart to choose life, abundant life!

My greatest desire is to lift Him up to His rightful place of honour, encouraging others along the way to experience the hope that is in Him alone.

4

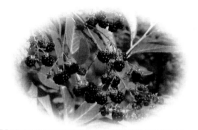

Humour

Life can mercilessly demand a serious side of us, threatening to overpower daily living. I experienced this challenge for the first year and a half following my accident. I was asked during one medical visit, "Kathie, what is it that you hope for most now that you have this disability?"

I remember replying, "To see the twinkle back in my eyes again. It's gone. I want it back."

Seeing pictures of myself at family gatherings after the accident was daunting. My eyes looked hollow and unexpressive, partly due to effects of the brain injury, but I also believe part of it was because I didn't know how to live anymore since acquiring my brain injury. I couldn't understand conversations, so joking and laughing was beyond my grasp. Others would laugh and I would force a smile, but inside I felt so robbed of this simple joy others could share with each other. I was also extremely overwhelmed as I tried desperately to keep up with everything that was taking place. The degree of fatigue I experienced was severe. The straightforward question really tugged at my heart and I knew something had to change. But how?

Humour always had a special role in my life. Getting or giving a giggle always provided a feather-filled lightness that just made everyone feel good. Humour makes a great day greater, a bad day brighter. It offers a pleasant reprieve from the weight of burdens which seem almost too much to bear at times.

One day, God led me directly to some tools which have made a tremendous difference in reducing noise levels. They are custom-moulded earplugs. They come in various shapes and thicknesses, depending on noise protection requirements. Often used in places of employment of an industrial nature, these noise-blockers provide hearing protection. Lighter versions are also available, used to filter out noise when sleeping, particularly when snoring problems make it difficult to go to sleep! A mould of my ears was taken at our local hearing centre, then shipped away. Within two weeks, I went back to the hearing centre where the fit was checked out carefully. These custom-made earplugs have been an absolute lifesaver for me! I wear them every day to filter out loud noises or certain pitches. I wear them to church, shopping, at gatherings, and anywhere that is noisy or has multiple audible stimuli.

Because of this discovery I am now able to attend more events, if even for a short period of time. I often wear them at home, particularly during the summer when sounds on the beach become overwhelming. They don't stop all the maze of words, but they do filter out certain pitches and background noise, adding enormous value to daily living. Should someone speak softly to me while I'm wearing them, I am not able to catch all that is being said. I may miss out on certain conversations, but for the most part I can participate in a variety of events again. However, there are times when I am not aware of someone speaking to me directly. This becomes a bit tricky sometimes, because someone may have spoken to me in a grocery store or somewhere else and I haven't heard them.

Unfortunately, some people don't realize I'm wearing earplugs. A time or two, someone has been offended because I didn't respond to their greeting, however I simply didn't realize anyone was talking to me. Ever learning, I try to combat that now by informing others of my need to wear earplugs quite often. I encourage them to tap me on the shoulder so I am aware of them, otherwise I may not respond. This adaptation has been an enormous blessing to me, opening new doors of opportunity, yet I have become much more aware of how challenging it must be for the hearing impaired and other disabled folks. Occasionally, when in a store brimming with noise and activity, I will ask for help. I let an employee know that I need to see their lips in order to understand them. They nod and smile, then turn their back to me, arms waving around as they chatter away while leading me to a specific area. I giggle now and patiently follow behind them. I just want to get what I need so I can get out of the store! Our society is so unaware of how to interact with people who have special needs.

Music has warmed my soul as long as I can remember. Our home, and my car, were filled with its beauty as if we depended on it to breathe. Experiencing the inability to enjoy music like I had previously felt like a huge deficit in my life. It was extremely difficult to accept.

Early one evening, following a discussion with precious friends regarding a chapter in the study book *A Purpose Driven Life* by Rick Warren, I asked our friend if he would play a song on his guitar, softly. My soul was craving the comfort and peace music often brings, particularly after sharing God's Word. I missed it so much. I hungered to lift my voice in song to the Lord, so I had asked our friend to bring his guitar. He pulled it out of its case and I popped in my "bugs," as I call them. Together the four of us, brothers and sisters in Christ, softly sang praises to our Lord and King.

It was a beautiful and cherished time enriched by loved ones who are constant and faithful companions. Their love is priceless and they provide tremendous encouragement and support for my newly acquired special needs. They personally know what it means to suffer from a disability, as his restricts their lives to some degree. We admire his courage and determination and we deeply cherish the common bond we share, loving our Lord Jesus Christ. His wife, one of my dearest friends, encourages and supports her sweetheart. Their marriage of thirty-plus years is a wonderful testament of unconditional love, for each other and for their Lord.

When we finished singing, he led our little group of four in prayer. At the end of the prayer he looked at me, hugged me, and with a twinkle in *his* eye, said, "I've never had anyone put earplugs in when I've played my guitar." We all burst into laughter as he joked how my earplugs were actually a compliment for his music, when in most cases it would make a musician question his talent! It was that innocent moment, when I heard the freedom of our laughter, that I grasped the robe of truth. My disability wasn't something to apologize for. That very special night, God changed something deep inside of me. I believe that was the first time since the accident that laughter erupted so freely.

Slowly, I began to start teasing others again. Understanding and acceptance were becoming more constant companions, and I was growing stronger in the realization that God has blessed my life *with life*. I began to ease up on my arduous focus toward the necessary parts of adapting. Initially, questions and uncertainties consumed me as I sought for answers and ways to cope. However, I had worked through the most difficult parts of grappling with the unknown. My intense but necessary homework had been done, opening a way to new horizons. The lighter side of life had begun to make its glorious reentrance.

Time can be our greatest friend, but only when coupled with patience. Much patience. Ecclesiastes 7:8–11 gives credence to the understanding of that truth: *"The end of a matter is better than its beginning, and patience is better than pride. Do not be quickly provoked in your spirit, for anger resides in the lap of fools. Do not say, 'Why were the old days better than these?' For it is not wise to ask such questions."*

Overcoming trials and challenges, growing in character, and surrendering to God are stepping stones which must be taken one at a time. In God's timing. His gentle, loving hand has been progressively opening up the treasure chest of gifts He has set aside for me. As I carefully sift through, I am beginning to experience deep-rooted joy in the discovery of my uniqueness. The treasures must be unwrapped one by one so each can be thoroughly accepted, enjoyed and used. He does not want me to take more than He is offering at one given time. It is the only way I can appreciate the fullness and value of each and every gift.

Right after the accident, humour, particularly spontaneous humour, was almost non-existent. Just trying to figure out life changes, humour didn't rate very high on my list and it seemed as though the accident had claimed humour as its victim as well. The serious side of life needed to be dealt with, and an enormous amount of energy was required to get through each day successfully. Failure often bit at my heels, and the close of the day seemed to offer no relief. I was confused, frustrated, frightened and overwhelmed with the stark reality that I could not handle many previous responsibilities anymore. The blanket of fatigue seemed to constantly cover me. Humour just didn't factor in to all the things I needed to think about.

Thankfully, a good night's sleep threw back the blanket of fatigue and discouragement each morning. I always woke up with anticipation for the new day. "Maybe today I'll be able to accomplish something I'm familiar with," I contemplated hopefully. Unfortunately, my morning routine was anything but routine. Once the day got underway, my limitations harshly reminded me of my losses. Thus, humour remained a stranger as reality crashed the party day in and day out. Weary of working incredibly hard to push through this cloud of disruption in my life, I didn't offer humour a chance to resurface—until that memorable night with our friends.

The sound of my laughter seemed strange. As spontaneous laughter erupted, I covered my mouth, surprised at how loud it sounded! Laughter had been silenced by the seriousness and confusion of my limitations for so long that it truly took me by surprise. That night, God used our close friends to lead me onto the next stepping stone. A priceless gift from God's treasure chest of life had been reopened, used again after a period of dormancy. What a refreshing release it was!

I understood and was dealing with most of the serious issues. It was very freeing to let loose again. There are still times when I don't fully grasp the significance of jokes, but I will ask someone to repeat them. If that does not seem appropriate, I will smile and enjoy the "happy" of the moment. Kip always enlightens me later on, often creating a humourous moment all to itself. I'm sure the joke is not always as funny as it was in the moment, but if I choose to indulge in the essence of the humour, it is still there. Or, I find sheer delight in Kip's interpretation! There are endless ways to embrace humour and fun which don't require speed in understanding. Rediscovery of humour has brought so much joy into my life again. Despite the fatigue that habitually continues, humour has opened the door to more spontaneity.

When very tired, I now find myself in a goofy mood instead of being weighed down by the challenges of the day. One night I hid in the dark while getting ready for bed. Kip came upstairs, but couldn't find me (we used to do this occasionally prior to the accident). He proceeded to search for me, but did so silently. I had forgotten he did that. I get so flustered knowing he's there, just standing and listening. He's a pro at this silly game we play. I end up giggling so much he doesn't need to do anything else. As a result, he's continued to be the unconquerable "winner," so far! Allowing myself freedom to do this again guarantees a good night's sleep as I drift off with a light heart instead of one burdened. I also deeply appreciate my husband's lighter side, as it produces the eventual eruption of laughter, an act which is very healthy for the soul.

I gave our son a whoopee cushion for his twentieth birthday, another sure sign that Mom is starting to be "Mom" again. On another occasion, Kip and I hid in some bushes, jumping out to scare a good friend of ours when he drove into the driveway. And, we sure did! I tend to forget, however, that playing a joke on another provides fair game for reciprocation!

As mentioned in a previous chapter, I literally got lost in our back orchard while walking one afternoon. When Kip arrived home I was exhausted, frustrated, nauseated and in tears. He wrapped his arms around me and said very seriously, "That's okay, honey. I'll just place a little blinky light on your shirt or jacket, and then I'll know where to find you." The visual picture of that in my head generated an outburst of giggles. Anticipating my reaction, his laughter added to mine, significantly easing the frustration.

A friend who lived on our property at the time (the fellow we scared) was concerned about that situation also. Only he could respond in this fashion, "Well Kath, if I had known you were sitting on the well about to pass out I would have brought out the wheelbarrow, thrown you in and hauled you back to the house." Deciphering that look of "seriousness" on his face for a moment, I once again visually pictured that scene, my arms and legs dangling over the sides, flopping around like a ragdoll. It created such a sense of silliness that we all giggled and laughed until happy tears rolled down my face.

The situation itself was very unsettling, so Kip told me to carry a cell phone, but finding humour in circumstances such as this enormously changes the focus. Humour gently softens frustration, leading to more clarity. It's a life-changing tool enabling me to shift my focus from the discouragement of what I can't do to a positive focus of finding workable solutions. I don't walk in a reverse pattern anymore, and every time I use the wheelbarrow I giggle when I envision myself inside being bumped along like a ragdoll toward the house by a special friend who can see the lighter side of life.

Not long ago, we were honoured with the visit of extremely precious friends. They had moved far away, obeying God's call to pastor another church. Our friendship has remained through thirteen years of distance, actually deepening due to the wonderful invention of email. I was so excited to see them and physically hug them! Furthermore, I could hardly wait to drink in the bountiful humour that would arrive with them.

Laughter had been returning with much more ease, yet there was a remnant of something inside of me which still prevented that twinkle in my eyes from fully returning. I was aware of that but could not explain why, nor did I understand why. I only knew that the one thing I told my physician I wanted to experience again was largely but not fully restored. *Until* we shared our first cup of tea with these cherished friends. The voices, the smiles, the warm familiarity. It was as if time had not separated us. Not long into our visit, laughter erupted and there *it* was—in complete and unbridled fullness, the long-awaited twinkle in my eyes shimmered! By the end of our first visit with them, Kip and I knew it had returned and tears of joy accompanied it.

Why during this time? How did these precious friends reach deep inside me and draw it to the surface? Was it because of the familiarity and special bond of friendship with folks I love deeply? Was it their absolute and open acceptance of me, as *me,* without any hesitant awkwardness? I don't know the answers; I only know that I instantaneously felt its return. I felt tremendous freedom with this couple. They had been a treasured part of our lives for many years. They did not personally witness the changes that took place in my life after the accident occurred, however they were aware of them as I shared my, and our, struggles with them openly.

Perhaps it was their outstretched arms the moment we connected as if time had not been lost between us. Perhaps it was because no strain or awkwardness existed. They were the same couple we enjoyed so many years ago and our time together was founded on who we all were, as friends. They were mindful and considerate of my limitations, yet I was still Kathie to them. There were no comparisons to things I used to do, and our conversations were uplifting, positive, encouraging and fulfilling. In addition there was humour, lots of humour. The more we visited the more laughter we enjoyed.

Our friend started snapping pictures. We quickly discovered he doesn't wait for folks to get their pose together. No, he just starts clicking, taking shot after shot after shot. What fun he had with that! What fun we all had with that! The results were goofy, silly, and hilarious photos! The ease of laughter was exhilarating and I felt the fullness of uninhibited laughter finally release from within!

I wasn't self-conscious about my disability with them, because it simply wasn't a factor in our friendship. They respected my new limitations, but they also provided enormous encouragement regarding the things I was accomplishing, loving and accepting me as the same woman they have known for almost two decades. Life brings changes to everyone's lives as the years pass. For some, the changes are more profound. Yet the core of who we are, particularly as believers in Christ Jesus, not only remains but deepens as we grow in our walk with Him. It is that spiritual bond which links us in a very special way with fellow Christians.

When viewing the pictures our friend had taken, tears literally rolled down my face. There was no mistaking it, the twinkle in my eyes had clearly returned. The fullness of laughter was alive and active in my soul again. God enabled the gifts of these precious friends to make another positive and dramatic change in my life. I will always be grateful to Him, and to them, for the enormous blessing of their love.

How *do* you adequately thank friends who bring out the very best in you, encourage you, and stand faithfully beside you? How do you ever say thank you to friends who help unwrap a part of you that has been lost or hidden through times of trials and heartache? The answer to those questions lies in the blessing of deep friendship. They gracefully accept your expression of gratitude and continue to be a source of strength in your life. The first release of laughter had begun after a bible study with close friends, liberating laughter to come more easily, more often. The final remnant was drawn out by close friends a couple of years later. Cherished friends like these exude the unconditional love of Jesus Christ, and relationships with them are priceless, unconditional and eternal.

Moments of fun, laughter and humour are just that, moments or dots of time. The crux of what life is all about will determine whether such moments hold temporary elation, or whether they are rooted in deep and lasting joy which comes only through a life grounded in Jesus Christ. I have no doubt where the revival of my laughter has come from.

As a believer in Christ, I want to shine for Him. I want to radiate true joy and fullness of life through my Lord Who gives me life. Genuine, lasting joy far outlasts the temporary experience of happiness. Happiness is fleeting, dependent on circumstances and things. Happiness touches only the very surface of our lives, vanishing when circumstances change or things lose their novelty.

Joy is deep, lasting and based on a life encompassed with God's peace. It is a constant, regardless of circumstances, not depending on superficial, temporary elation. It does not shatter when life hits hard. God's vibrant gift of joy flows from within a soul craving something more eternal, something with more essence to it. Joy settles deeply into the heart of one who seeks Christ's Presence. It's there when life is light and, more importantly, when life seems unbearable. This is what lasting joy means to me: J-O-Y: **Jesus Overflowing in You!**

I really love to laugh, and I have grown in self-confidence, which empowers me to laugh easily at myself. I don't always say what I mean to say, particularly when I am really tuckered or at the close of the day, my "concentration" medication having worn off. Instead of saying "rag-a-muffin" I may come out with something like "mag-a-ruffin." My words are not always appropriate and it has caused moments of silence resulting in puzzled looks, including my own. I do not realize what has slipped out until a few seconds later, the processing of information finally reaching my internal "message board." After these honest malfunctions of the tongue, I often begin to giggle at what I've said. Although silence and odd looks may take place when this happens, others either join me, or the conversation ends.

Plastic spiders and other insects of the dollar-store kind *mysteriously* find their way into nooks and crannies of our home and property. They are very effective in their purpose. A good sense of humour is contagious and I find myself taken by surprise at times when they are planted by the one who had originally been the object of my schemes. The mischief which runs through my blood was inherited from my mother. When our children were little she would sneak a black, leggy spider under the covers of their beds or next to their cereal bowls before they headed off to school. What fun we had when she came to visit!

At times, I may misunderstand something which has been said due to a lot of activity or conversation. Trying to converse intellectually, I might say something quite unrelated to the topic at hand. Greater understanding of the way my brain functions has enabled me to relax more. I giggle and just let it pass, if others will let it pass.

Not long ago, I responded to a friend's comment by saying, "I know you know it all." My intent was to let my friend know I agreed with their thoughts about being knowledgeable in a certain area. They really did know what they were talking about, and I appreciated their candour in sharing that with me. A few seconds later, I realized it sounded like I was perhaps being sarcastic, that they *"knew it all."* That was not what I *meant* to express and that led to trying to remove the foot of inappropriate wording out of my mouth, which only made things worse. Fortunately my friend knows me well and responded with a humourous comeback, generating open and easy laughter. Good friends and family often don't let me off the hook easily anymore, and that stimulates the lighter side of life.

Humour is settling into its rightful place in my life once again. I know my twinkle is back and I know my wit is following closely behind. My "forever" friend who moved away a few years ago said to me as we chatted by telephone, "Oh Kath, it is *so* good to hear you laugh again!"

Thank you, Lord, for it *is* good to laugh again!

5

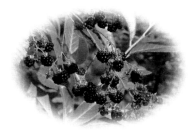

Problems X Answers = Victory!

Problems. A word I don't much care for. Complaining. Another word I have an aversion to. However, they do have a definitive place in our vocabulary. Over the years, I've tried to seek out ways to reduce their influence on my life. During this search I have come to the conclusion that for every problem there *is* a solution, even if it's not the solution our hearts were hoping for.

I've sought different ways to tackle whatever problem may come my way. Through trial and error, I've often waded through the sluggish mud of disappointment trying to find the solution to a particular problem. I've persisted, experiencing difficulties and challenges yet determined not to succumb to the point of becoming immovable or swallowed up. I've discovered that there are solutions to combat failure and mistakes. Recognizing that you have made a mistake is the first point in moving forward. I have at times pursued the wrong choices, and consequence bit at my heels; however, it was important to seek positive solutions to perceived dead ends. I yearned for growth even when it meant assuming risk by following through with a decision with no guarantee of success.

The quest for solid, workable solutions demands effort, time and patience. Ideally, a lot of prayer is involved, coupled with a willingness to heed God's guidance. Searching for workable answers to problems requires personal investment on my part, yet the victory of overcoming a problem is so rewarding that I am finally coming to a point of understanding how character is truly developed through the challenges. Continual efforts to work through, then beyond, problems prevent me from becoming stagnant. Beyond that, I am then in a healthy position to reach out to others who experience similar challenges.

I don't ever want to look into another person's eye as they go through heartache and pain only to insinuate they need a little more faith for things to work out the way they hope. Life's challenges don't always work out the way we hope they will, regardless of how much faith we possess. Sometimes we can be misguided as Christians, placing harsh judgment on our own spiritual walk or another's because valley after valley of struggle and heartache are experienced.

Complete surrender of our lives to the Lord Jesus Christ does not guarantee all we have planned for will work out as we anticipate. We won't always understand why things happen the way they do. Yet our Father requires us to have absolute faith in His leading. He knows every one of our mistakes and failures, but also the sincerity of our hearts as we desire to honour Him with our lives. When we surrender to Him, He will redeem the mistakes and failures. Beyond that blessing, He will open doors and windows of potential solutions that are ours to investigate.

My own heartaches and battles have opened my eyes and my heart to empathize with the depth of pain in another's life. I may question why certain circumstances take place, but I am learning not to question God's loyalty and faithfulness. Circumstances are ever-changing, God is unchanging. Grasping this spiritual truth has prepared me to face them straight on. Often it is His strength that carries me when my own fails miserably, the trial and heartache at hand overwhelming me.

Each person is unique and no one can ever truly know what it is like to walk in another person's shoes. The road gets bumpy, very bumpy at times, but steadfast friends and family unquestionably help smooth out the rougher spots, especially if they have struggled along their own bumpy path.

A friend and former employee called me a while ago. Having been in a car accident a few years ago, she now experiences challenges similar to my own. She shared how she had tried so hard to understand my newly imposed limitations and frustrations during the initial years following my accident. She thought she had gained a pretty good understanding of the situation, until she was in an accident herself. Through different eyes, she now sees why it had been so difficult for me to work, socialize or just get through each day. She has utilized some of my adaptations and she enquired about some solutions I have implemented. It is now personal, so despite her struggles to deal with injuries, she *will* be a blessing to others. She is growing, too.

God is really clear in His Word that He will never give us more than we can bear. In Psalm 145:13–14 David declares, *"… The LORD is faithful to all his promises, and loving toward all he has made. The LORD upholds all those who fall and lifts up all who are bowed down."* Personally, that translates into the following: When I fall spiritually, emotionally or otherwise, God will always lift me up with His strong, yet gentle and loving hands. He will provide all I need to carry on as I strive to fulfill His purpose for my life, fixing my eyes upon Him.

This is why He created me in the first place—to serve Him, making Him Lord of my life. I was created to bring God pleasure resulting in the fulfillment of His purpose for my life. I was also designed for intimate communion and fellowship with Him. If He permitted life to coast along with no problems or challenges, what on earth would I need Him for? How often would I really commune with Him in an intimate manner? How many times would He cross my mind in any given day?

Life does get tough and we are tested unbearably at times. This testing does not always come from God; it can be prompted by Satan, with God's permission. This is evident in the book of Job. Job experienced Satan's ruthlessness, yet his faith in God was absolute, despite insurmountable losses. God ultimately remained in control. He also remained unconditionally faithful to Job.

Sin and its consequences can also initiate times of brutal testing, challenging our faith and our obedience to God's Holy Word. We often want to do things our way, pushing the will of God aside. Yet He remains close, only a whisper away until we realize the destruction our own will has brought upon us. When we genuinely repent our inward focus, God will guide us through the adversity of ill-made decisions.

Yes, God promises to carry us when burdens weigh heavily upon our shoulders. He promises to remain right by our side even when we become strong enough to walk on our own again. He is forever faithful, providing wisdom, knowledge and understanding, at His discretion. My responsibility is to do everything I know how to do, surrendering the rest to Him to deal with supernaturally. I have the power of the Holy Spirit within to hand over the "chicken plate" to Him.

Tremendous, unfathomable freedom destroys prison bars of doubt, fear, uncertainty and worry when we place our trust in Him, not ourselves. My inner confidence that God lovingly answers prayer in a way only He can, binds my heart to His, substantiating an unshakable trust in Him. I rely heavily on my Heavenly Father's help, and I need His guidance every step of the way. This especially holds true for wavering emotions and internal struggles which challenge a focused walk.

On one particular occasion, I heard someone suggest that leaning on God through difficult times was "just a crutch," a display of weakness. Well then, let's examine what purpose a crutch fulfills? When in use it offers strength, healing, mobility, ease of pain as it reduces pressure, and much more freedom to stay involved in life's activities. Leaning on God offers strength, healing, stability in my life, and ease of emotional pain as He reduces pressure. My symbolic crutch is made from a tree on which my Saviour died for me. His unconditional love, forgiveness and grace provide spiritual restoration for my soul, just as a tangible crutch provides physical restoration to a broken leg. He loves me so much He was willing to be crucified, dying a horrible death as He took upon Himself the weight of my sin, your sin and the sins of the entire world. He was crudely left to hang on a cross made out of wood. But His death was not the end.

There is more, so much more. The empty cross is a powerful reminder of the depth of our Father's love, and it holds incredible promise for me, and you. Christ's barbaric death ultimately led to His victorious resurrection, offering eternal life to all who believe. My symbolic crutch enables me to walk along the *only* road leading to eternal life. Spiritual restoration is eternal. Quite some crutch, isn't He?

Reliance on God is critical to life-changing success, but I must take the necessary steps to personally be proactive. I am required to do all that I can do. God's expectation for us to respond proactively to the work He has called us to do is illustrated throughout His Word. When we have an intimate relationship with Him, He will always require obedience from us.

There are so many examples to draw from, but one of the simplest yet most profound comes from Mary, the mother of Jesus. God chose her to fulfill His purpose of delivering the Messiah to save the world. Out of the entire human race on earth at that time, He chose her. Opening our Bibles more than two thousand years later, we may presume that this would be an honour of the highest calling. For Mary it was—she trusted God completely. Culturally, however, disgrace and the possibility of being stoned was the reality she faced, not honour. I can't begin to imagine the questions, fear and doubt that must have washed over this young virgin. How could this transpire when she was still a virgin? Would Joseph her beloved believe her? How would they deal with the strict customs of the times as far as marriage was concerned? Chapters one and two in the Book of Luke provide a brief glimpse of the feelings that enveloped Mary.

Despite the uncertainty at hand with no foreknowledge as to what the future would hold, she completely trusted God and did everything He instructed her to do. Mary willingly yielded to God. Luke 1:38 reveals her response to the angel bearing the news: *"'I am the Lord's servant,' Mary answered. "May it be to me as you have said.'"* Immediately, in reverential obedience, she and Joseph prepared to do what God instructed them to do. There was so much for them to discuss, yet their trust in Him was uninhibited.

He expects that of me, disability and all. Humbly, I seek His will. I want to respond as His servant to the call He has placed before me. He has a unique purpose for my life and He wants me to use all that He has given me. He wants me to obey His leading without reservation. I can release the rest to Him, trusting in His power and strength to do what I cannot. I allow Him to be Who He is: God! Almighty! Powerful! Yes, He wants me to pursue solutions that align with His guidance, and He expects me to act on them. I need to be proactive. It is my responsibility to do my homework, exploring alternatives and concrete solutions for problems and challenges that frequently arise. Digging deep inside for determination and strength to overcome challenges enables me to grow steadfast in spirit and character by accepting challenges straightforwardly instead of buckling under them or trying to simply avoid them.

The Bible tells us in Ephesians 2:10, *"For we are God's workmanship, created in Christ Jesus to do good works, which God prepared in advance for us to do."* God has a whole itinerary for me to work through. In fact, as the Scripture above clearly states, He has prepared this for me, in advance. He has placed such confidence in me that He has already prepared things for me to do. Paul does not add a clause saying, "Unless circumstance or disability prevents further progress." The accident was not a surprise to God; He knew of it long before I did. His plans for me are still laid out, and it is my task to discover what they are so I can proceed. It is crucial to remember He will never place anything into my life which He and I cannot handle together.

I have only recently had the courage to look back to assess what has transpired since the accident. God's hand is clearly visible as He patiently and lovingly leads me through this new journey. In my growth I am unearthing healthy and positive solutions, empowering me to work through the many difficulties I have experienced, and will continue to experience. I've leaned heavily on His guidance, sometimes stumbling as I try to decipher His answers. I don't always know if I am doing things correctly, therefore communion with Him is essential.

He is quick to let me know if I am on the right track or if I need to change direction. He will open the door wider or He will close it. Because of my relationship with Him, I can stand secure in His guidance. I may have to be patient, waiting until He is ready to reveal His will to me. Sensitivity to His leading bestows confidence to experiment with different adaptations until I figure out what works best. I believe He is guiding that process so I can discern His purpose for my life.

Failure in trying is success in the making. Sometimes I still try to tackle things which are too far-reaching for me. Do I then give up, tossing the entire challenge to the wind? Not for a minute! Alternatively, I'll take a smaller bite, which allows me to peek through the door of possibility. Success may still be attainable, but it may come in a different package than I had originally anticipated. Following the accident, I decided to enroll in a quilting 101 class. My sewing knowledge was basic, but I felt the instructional process and classroom setting would help me reclaim former capabilities. I had a rude awakening. Short-term memory loss, confusion and a processing shortfall were harsh representatives of my new limitations. I tried to persevere with the classes, but to no avail. The instructors were wonderful, offering accessibility as needed. Despite intense headaches and turtle-paced progress, I did eventually finish the wall quilt at home.

Several years later, I began creating my own, small projects. Calculating measurements and having to mentally visualize a project definitely stimulates and challenges my brain. I am able to work at my own pace, and a healthy sense of accomplishment washes over me when another project is complete and ready to give to someone special.

Through trial and error, I have encountered deeper contentment and satisfaction with the progress in my life. Frustration doesn't rob my optimism for solutions anymore. Persistent efforts to do my best, whether viewed as successful by others or not, is producing personal confidence, thus holding great promise for all the tomorrows still ahead of me.

Satan, the father of lies, will go to great lengths to steal the victory banner from our hold. We will find the world's perception of victory drastically different from God's, but I firmly believe that any time we obey God's leading and guidance, we can stand secure in God's winner's circle. David speaks of the certainty we can claim in Psalm 37:23–24, *"If the LORD delights in a man's way, he makes his steps firm; though he stumble, he will not fall, for the LORD upholds him with his hand."* What greater assurance of victory could there possibly be? Colossians 3:23–24 instructs, "*Whatever you do, work at it with all your heart, as working for the Lord, not for men, since you know that you will receive an inheritance from the Lord as a reward. It is the Lord Christ you are serving.*"

"Well done, good and faithful servant!" These are the most glorious words anyone could ever hear from the Lord. Fulfilling God's plan for our lives through a genuine desire to serve Jesus Christ is all He asks of us. To seek Him when problems arise, to praise Him when blessings abound, and to ordain Him as our ultimate Guide as we tread along life's pathway. "Well done, good and faithful servant." Victory in any other form could never be nearly as sweet!

PART SIX

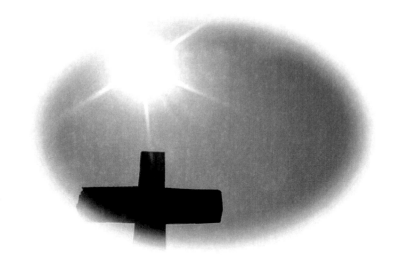

WORTHY—BY GOD'S SAVING GRACE ALONE

*"For he chose us in him before the creation of the world to be holy
and blameless in his sight. In love he predestined us to be adopted as his
sons through Jesus Christ, in accordance with his pleasure and will—to the
praise of his glorious grace, which he has freely given us in the One he loves.
In him we have redemption through his blood, the forgiveness of sins, in
accordance with the riches of God's grace that he lavished on us
with all wisdom and understanding."*
(Ephesians 1:4–8)

Photo © 2006 Kris K.W. Pritchard

1

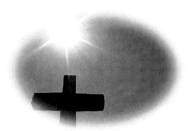

PASSION

WHOLEHEARTEDLY JUMPING INTO LIFE IS PART OF MY CHARACTER AND personality. It's a large part of what makes me tick. This trait has continued to hold true since my accident as I have tried diligently to work through the encircling confusion generated by my disability, determined to overcome. Perhaps at times my tenacity has augmented the intensity of my frustrations. My limitations hindered me, but my spirit was determined to win the battle. Defeat wasn't an option I had any interest exploring. Nevertheless, even my determined spirit could not prevent, fix or have power over the encumbering effects of my disability.

From the very depth of my heart, I sought to regain wholeness of personal well-being, a wholeness strongly embedded in my spirit. However, restoration of its strength was another story. Physical changes had taken place within my body and within the processing area of my brain. The first year had been a mass of confusion, turmoil, pain, anger, frustration and emotional upheaval. I couldn't pinpoint what was wrong with me. I often felt I was banging against an unseen wall every time I tried to move forward. I could not see around or through it.

Days, weeks, and months passed by. I began to realize there was no other alternative but to make a deliberate choice to destroy this wall, or be consumed by it. It was becoming emblematic of the difficulties and limitations my disability presented, at the present time and into the future. I didn't like the direction I was heading, with uncertainty and constant "failures" weighing me down heavily. My heart sought God's guidance. Psalm 31:24 challenged me, *"Be strong and take heart, all you who hope in the LORD."* He alone would be my beacon of hope to regain wholeness of life once again. Only He could guide me as I fumbled to find an opening in what seemed to be an impenetrable wall of doubt.

Physically, I struggled with exhaustion, mental fatigue, confusion, nausea, headaches and shoulder pain. Tiring quickly from simple activities robbed much of the motivation and means to fully experience the same zest for life. I battled between the fiery desire of wanting my energy back and the stark reality of its absence. That passion for life which surfaced so naturally prior to the accident had become extremely difficult, if not impossible at times, to resurrect.

I was told repeatedly by professionals to stay within the boundaries of my newly acquired disability or discouragement would gain ground. I desperately wanted to "gain ground," but in a positive direction, not wanting to constantly slip on a downward slope toward defeat. Despite their stern warnings, these professionals also offered constant encouragement. There was also someone else Who could truly help me succeed, someone Who was accessible at all times, even when I sought counsel with a small, whispering voice in the dead of night.

Walking daily with the Lord meant He was right by my side. When I stumbled and slipped, I knew He would stand firmly, His powerful hand outstretched to pull me forward. It was up to me to grasp my Father's outstretched hand so He could safely lift me to level ground again. His proven faithfulness intensified my resolve to focus once again on the path before me. God's Holy Word promises He is faithfully beside us at all times. He doesn't always eliminate our challenges, but He does remain faithful with an outstretched arm when our strength wanes. Psalm 18:31–33 says, *"For who is God besides the LORD? And who is the Rock except our God? It is God who arms me with strength and makes my way perfect. He makes my feet like the feet of a deer; he enables me to stand on the heights."* Only through my surrendered heart's search of these precious promises did He revitalize my resolve to continue the upward climb.

There was no advantage in looking backward to analyze what I was leaving behind. The focus needed to be different now in order for me to regain wholeness of life and that necessitated adherence to my newly acquired limits. I began to understand how absolute wholeness of life comes through acceptance of who we are in Jesus Christ. My energy level began to respond favourably to healthy boundaries I started implementing, thus reawakening my passion for life from its place of slumber.

Passion for life enhances life regardless of circumstances, but it must be allowed to flow naturally from the well of balanced living. I did not want this disability to suppress my passionate spirit. I knew God had given me my zest for life, and I had to trust He would never desire to take that away. I had to be completely willing and open in order for the Holy Spirit to move in me, and through me. This process enlightened me as to the importance of patience and the wisdom of waiting for direction.

Times of helplessness definitely toyed with my focus, but I do not recall ever suffering the oppression of utter hopelessness. I perceive this to be one of those quiet but powerful miracles resulting from my awareness of direct access to the Lord God Almighty, my Creator. Regardless of my feelings while conversing with Him, He has always protected me from hopelessness. I refuse to surrender to Satan's lies, murmurs of how life will never be as full as it used to be. It will never *be* as it used to be, but through God's power and my passion to live abundantly in this God-given life, the new journey begins. Satan's murmurs become mumbled nonsense.

I saw my precious mother climb mountains which seemed impossible to conquer. Her faith and dependence on Christ was unwavering. I grew up in a home where joy did not depend on glorious, perfect circumstances. Through her daily example, particularly during my formative years, I witnessed firsthand how true, deep, and lasting joy filled her soul, a direct result of Christ having first place in her heart. Young eyes silently absorb what is often unseen to others. I understood at a very tender age that to live passionately for Him was to give Him my entire being. It meant trusting lock, stock and barrel that He would use this willing vessel to do His intended work. I was aware there may be tears, questions, and frustration during the journey. Yet the most important truths rose above all of that. God is faithful and compassionate. He is Lord.

My personal elucidation of those truths is profoundly engrained in me. I cannot and will not exchange them for lies whispered from the father of lies who cowers in darkness, terrified to see the Light of Truth. Satan can never come close to matching the fullness of life our Holy Father, God Almighty, promises His beloved children. Never.

People watch how we live for Christ, particularly when we proclaim Him as Lord and Saviour. Factitious magnifying glasses are often slipped on to examine a life that proclaims Christ as Lord. When tragedy or suffering occurs, internal questions surface: "Will they still love and trust their God the same way now?"

Our love affair with God requires an unselfish commitment to accept His will, even when His will is difficult to decipher or understand. It involves trusting Him completely, regardless of circumstances. I have questioned myself, "What does my life reveal *now*? Does His glory shine through even this?" Psalm 40:1–3 says, *"I waited patiently for the LORD; he turned to me and heard my cry. He lifted me out of the slimy pit, out of the mud and mire; he set my feet on a rock and gave me a firm place to stand. He put a new song in my mouth, a hymn of praise to our God. Many will see and fear and put their trust in the LORD."*

What amazing promises David reflects on in this passage! God reveals the depth to which He is committed to us through those promises. He also requires something from us. We are to be proactive in this personal relationship with Him. First, I need to wait patiently. Those two words combined almost seem an oxymoron! Wait. Patiently. It is so hard just to wait for anything sometimes, let alone answers to significant questions about life itself! Surely the Lord sees how much I want to move forward, progress and be proactive! Yet David tells us that he had to wait, patiently. He was obviously in a place of frustration and turmoil. The same instructions apply to us. God doesn't want me to complain while I wait, nor does He want me to demand that He hurry up. He instructs me to wait patiently for His guidance.

It is only God who knows the individual and personal challenges I will face, and only He knows the hurdles I will have to jump over. Trusting in His Omnipotent Supremacy, I depend on Him to carry me through. He designed a plan for my life and He knows the pathway I must walk. Each step must not be rushed. He is the author of my life and if He tells me to wait for His guidance, then I must wait. Patiently. Secondly, He promises He will *turn* toward me. He will reach out His hand and He will help me. Each time I have fallen, He has tenderly gathered the broken pieces, restoring my life to fullness again. As I hold tightly to His hand, He gently leads me in the direction He wants me to go. I do not have to struggle on my own!

There will always be circumstances that test my spirit, but I don't have to be afraid of slipping or losing my grip in the mud only to fall even deeper into the quicksand of darkness and despair. God promises He will rescue me from that place of distress. More astounding than that, God the Father will then place my feet on a solid rock, giving me security and confidence in who I am in Him. Praising Him passionately comes easily when I open my eyes to the miracles He is blessing my life with. Powerful words contained within the stanzas of a much-loved hymn testify to this specific promise of God. *"On Christ the solid rock I stand, all other ground is sinking sand. All other ground is sinking sand."*

I pray that those watching what is taking place in my life, and in my marriage, will clearly recognize God's power. I pray many will take hold of how very real and personal He is. Imperfection, mistakes, errors in judgment, and sin—whether intentional or otherwise—unashamedly remind me of my human weakness. I've made many mistakes, most resulting from my own stubbornness and will, and He has lovingly disciplined me just as any caring Father would. Truthfully, perfection is something only God can lay claim to. Yet through the blood of Jesus, genuine repentance brings redemption, and my canvas of life is wiped clean to begin anew. My relationship with Christ is something I have never been ashamed of, but along with that intimate relationship comes great responsibility to uphold His commands. I don't always succeed. I am very aware of the glass house I now live in, knowing my life will or will not give witness to the power of God's involvement. My walk with Him must be genuine so His Holy Spirit can work through me and within me.

God never pulls away from us; however, we draw away from Him at times. Even so, He remains forever close, patiently waiting for us to invite Him onto the throne of our hearts once again. He doesn't push, nag, intrude or ridicule. He waits patiently. He wants us to come to Him because of our deep love for Him. We are not puppets on a life-string that He manipulates. He has created us with the dignity of freedom to make our own choices. His heart overflows with delight when we place our entire lives into His care for safekeeping.

God's unwavering faithfulness and amazing grace are what keep our relationship so personal. I fervently pray that the joy, faithfulness, confidence and passion I've experienced because of His life-changing power will be silently observed. I do not need to know, nor is it my place to know, who may receive Christ as their personal Saviour because I have allowed God to use me, mould me and fill me. My role is to live for Him, shine for Him and declare Him as Lord. His gift to me is a deep, unexplainable, lifelong peace and the reward of eternal life with Him.

It may seem easier to believe in God when life is coasting along comfortably, but the victory of reassurance and underlying peace in the midst of a traumatic event cannot be matched when it is the direct result of a personal relationship with Jesus Christ. The true assessment of my faith, especially during adversity, reveals my commitment to and unwavering trust in the One I proclaim as Lord.

As a result of this accident and my newly acquired disability, my path has crossed with many people I would have never otherwise met. God has been present in all interactions and I have felt His Holy Spirit with me. I have been able to share God's strength, guidance and faithfulness as I've talked with many doctors, specialists and other professionals over the past few years. I simply cannot remain silent about the incredible role He fulfills in my life! I love Him so passionately! He is so genuinely real and there is not one area of my life not cared for or directed by Him!

My faith has grown tremendously as I've witnessed God at work in my life. Matthew 12:34 says, *"For out of the overflow of the heart the mouth speaks."* This passage speaks of discipline in what we say, but it can also present other food for thought. Out of the overflow of love in my heart for Christ, I passionately share what He is doing in my life, any way I can! Knowing Christ cares for me in such an intimate way makes my heart soar. I get so excited to share what God is doing in my life because my heart is so full of love for Him! He wants us to enjoy life, not just endure it! How awesome to be able to praise Him from sunrise to sunset!

Sometimes my faith is not understood or accepted. Sometimes I am told I am not being "realistic." However, living with Jesus as my Lord and Saviour, knowing how intimate and real He truly is, makes it impossible for me to see things any other way! I know what I'm living and I know Who is giving me abundant life!

As mentioned throughout these pages, this does not mean I will never stumble. Loving Him with every part of who I am does not eliminate all of my shortcomings. I still make mistakes, I still stumble and fall, and I still do wrong things and make bad decisions. I struggle periodically with self-doubt, and disheartening wounds still fester when I wrestle with certain issues that should have been released to God. When that happens, it's a good time to take stock. I usually discover I have temporarily turned my back to God during those periods, in order to figure something out on my own. He has not let me out of His sight or care; rather it is I who chose to take my focus off Him.

But it is that disquieting recognition of my sin and periodic waywardness which brings to the forefront the very reason I celebrate my relationship with the Trinity! Humbly going before God, with a genuine heart of repentance for pursuing my will instead of His, results in His forgiveness and cleansing of my soul. Through the blood of Jesus Christ, His one and only Son, I am renewed. Forgiven, I become clean once again. My heart is no longer stained and it sparkles with promise for being used once again by God!

God discloses how He wants me to live through His Word, The Holy Bible. He shows me what I am to do to remain in accordance with His will. Each time I fall into sin, I must genuinely ask for cleansing. True repentance comes from a deep-rooted sorrow within my heart for hurting my Lord. It also means consciously turning from that sin, determined not to do it again. By God's saving grace and Christ's complete atonement for my sin through His death on the cross, I am forgiven and my heart becomes clean once again.

I often said to our children as they were growing, "When we genuinely ask forgiveness from Jesus, our sin is thrown into the sea of forgetfulness. He remembers it no more." Fresh, brand new steps are ours to walk the moment we seek God's forgiveness. The Holy Spirit then fills our entire being with the freedom that is found only through the blood of Jesus Christ. The dirt gets left behind, wiped away for good. This offer is open to every human being on this entire planet. He is only, *only* a prayer away. The difference He makes in each individual life is beyond comprehension. His gift of abundant life and eternal life is absolutely free and can never be bought or earned. Christ paid the ultimate price for us and we have complete and glorious victory in the fullness of life which comes from our personal relationship with Him. It is our responsibility to unwrap the gift, embracing its eternal value.

We all get excited over something profound that occurs in our lives. Every single person does. Believer and non-believer. We can hardly wait to share *our* story. When Christ fills our entire being with Himself, how can we contain our joy? Our confidence in Him? Our worth in Him? Some will yearn to experience the joy, the passion. Some will not understand it and others will reject it altogether. But when this holy freedom is personally and intimately experienced, rivers of joy flow ceaselessly from the life in whom He resides. Colossians 2:6–7 says, *"So then, just as you received Christ Jesus as Lord, continue to live in him, **rooted** and built up in him, strengthened in the faith as you were taught, and **overflowing with thankfulness**"* (emphasis mine). How exciting to passionately live for Jesus!

2

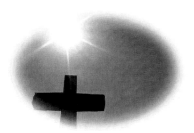

MIRACLES

LEARNING TO LET GO OF THE DESIRE TO ACCESS ABILITIES I NO LONGER possess has produced an overwhelming need to explore the truth about miracles. I have always believed in God-given miracles and I know wonderful and miraculous miracles do take place.

There has been much prayer for God to heal me, and at times I have personally wondered why He hasn't. Maybe if I prayed harder. Maybe if I read my Bible more or had more faith. Yet God in His mercy and grace asks not that I try to muster up more faith to "believe more," but rather that I step back and look at what is taking place in my life, right now. When our eyes fix (completely focus) on Him, He removes self-focus, replacing it with spiritual eyes that look to Him for answers to the questions asked. His Holy Word unveils wonderful truths about the power of tangible miracles, many of these performed by our Lord Jesus. So what do I see? How do these biblical revelations apply to my life? Partly through Scripture and partly through prayer, I began to recognize the glorious wonder of miracles which take place deep within the heart even when no physical miracle of healing takes place.

I believe I am discovering the peace, joy and even pure delight in everyday miracles which far surpass holding out for the big one. Our Lord God declares in Isaiah 43:18–19, *"Forget the former things; do not dwell on the past. See, I am doing a new thing! Now it springs up; do you not perceive it?"* Wow! I get *very* excited about this area of faith. I do believe that God alone has complete and infinite power to divinely heal our bodies physically, if that is what He wills. However, I also believe our expectations and personal human definitions of what it means to be healed are often very different from what God intends to do supernaturally with the life He has created. His focus is outward, toward us. Our focus is inward, to what we want to receive.

Most of the time, seeking miracles from Almighty God generally means that we request or state to God what *we* want to see happen. God does tell us to ask for anything in His name, to lay our requests before Him. This spurs us on to make requests of Him, even of a divine nature. Yet voicing those requests, even quietly, requires great steps of faith and trust as we expose our vulnerability, heartaches and weaknesses, pleading for healing, for wholeness to return. Requesting this from Him with an unguarded heart is the first step toward true healing, whether physical or spiritual.

At times it is within God's plan to heal physically in the miraculous way we have requested, and anticipated. Much praise and glory is lifted up to Him from tremendously grateful and thankful hearts. However, there are many times when it appears as though God does not hear, or respond. We fall despondent, despairing because He has not done what we have literally begged of Him to do. He seems to be silent. It's as though He has turned away. But has He? Or have we been so humanly focused on requesting a specific form of healing that we become blind to the healing He wants to take place in us? What I perceive to be a miracle may not be in God's plan for my life at all. When asking for a miracle, I find myself often requesting something I deeply desire because I believe it is something I, or someone else needs. Many loving people have prayed for miracles to take place in my life to restore what

I have lost, so I can be the person I used to be, so I can be "whole" again.

The love that flows from the hearts behind these genuine prayers deeply touches me. They are sincere, loving and brought before God in faith. Yet I continue to have limitations imposed by my disability. Subsequent to my accident, the absence of physical healing seemed to suggest unanswered or perhaps unheard prayer. I wondered why God would choose not to heal me. I wondered why He was not answering prayers, mine or others. I love Him deeply and, though far from perfect, I try to be obedient to His Word. Was I doing something wrong to prevent His healing?

Searching for truth and answers can turn into a wonderful exploration of God's heart. The definition of the word miracle as found in the Oxford Dictionary says, "An extraordinary and welcome event believed to be the work of God...a remarkable and very welcome occurrence..."

My questions began to take a different form as God patiently disclosed His truths once again. My life was created for His purpose, not my own. I began to ask myself if I was really open to the possibility that miracles were already taking place. Perhaps it would not be the "big" physical miracle which I and others had pleaded for, the miracle that would visibly restore my body and mind, reestablishing me as the familiar, comfortable Kathie I had been before the accident.

That was what I willed for. What I desired relied on the assumption that God's answer would surely be in accordance with my will. But what if the miracle(s) I sought were not in line with God's will for my life? What if He desired something completely different to fulfill a purpose of great importance to Him? A purpose I was not yet aware of? I had never explored that possibility.

It did not occur to me that God may not want the "old" Kathie reestablished. 2 Corinthians 5:17 states, *Therefore, if anyone is in Christ, he is a new creation; the old has gone, the new has come!*" This passage refers to the rebirth of new life when we die to our old selves, sin and all. Spiritually reborn, we become vibrantly fresh, new and changed inside as we choose to walk in the Light of our Lord and Saviour, Jesus Christ. This new life does not stop at conversion. It is available every moment of every day we walk with our Lord. And this new life is open to every human being, disabled or not.

This revelation brought about a renewed focus in my chats with Him. I began to ask for His will to be done in my life. I want to walk on the pathway of life that He has chosen for me, because it will be the only pathway to fullness in this life. A life under the personal care of the Great Physician brings a calming sense of inner peace. God removes blinders from our eyes when we read His Word with sincere and seeking hearts. He provides understanding on a much deeper level than the world can offer.

I am beginning to experience God's power in a way I never have before. My entire life I have loved Jesus and trusted Him. There have been times when struggles encamped around Kip and me, and we turned to Him for divine guidance. He never let us down. However, we had never been tested to this degree before. My brain injury is something that cannot be fixed, or changed. The necessity to learn a new way of living has provided much greater, life-changing challenges. Attempting to do that alone has not ever been an option for either of us.

Gradual acceptance that God has allowed my disability to remain has enabled my heart to recognize, and embrace, the blessings His Holy Spirit is bringing into my life and the lives of others daily. When we seek we will find answers, albeit different answers perhaps from those we anticipated. Only by completely surrendering our personal requests while seeking God's answers can we begin to confidently identify how He is choosing to work in our lives. A continual hunger draws me in to God's Word daily. God could have done things differently at the time of the accident, yet He chose to allow this particular turn in the pathway. Acknowledging that grants me the freedom and desire to see what He wants to do with my life, what He will do, and ultimately where He will lead. The words of Oswald Chambers challenge me in such a healthy way. He said, "Beware of harking back to what you were once when God wants you to be something you have never been."[3]

Through the ensuing years, persistent challenges of my disability will allow me the privilege of conferring with Him daily. It will allow His

---

[3] Oswald Chambers, *My Utmost for His Highest*, 1963, with permission.

magnificent power to reign in my life. That statement probably sounds peculiar, but that is how I choose to view the future. The disability is permanent, that fact remains. How I choose to handle it makes all the difference in the world, because my decision will determine the value and quality of the years ahead. I can face the future holding His hand, depending on Him, optimistic about proactively participating in the exciting journey ahead with Him. Or I can struggle and battle aimlessly through a foggy pathway without God, dragging my physical limitations behind me along with the heavier and destructive burdens of resentment, bitterness, and anger.

Psalm 105:4 says, *"Look to the LORD and his strength; seek his face always."* John 3:30 says, *"He must become greater; I must become less."* I expect God to fulfill His promises. Through His Word, I commune with Him daily for guidance and wisdom. Prayerfully, I seek the ability to recognize the things He requires me to do, releasing the things I can't to Him for supernatural intervention. This is thrilling! Psalm 37:5–7 says, *"Commit your way to the LORD; trust in him and he will do this; He will make your righteousness shine like the dawn, the justice of your cause like the noonday sun. Be still before the LORD and wait patiently for him."* I absolutely love this passage. First command? Commit my life's journey to the Lord. This involves surrender and submission. It is not a derogatory command, but rather a supportive one.

Sincere commitment, surrender and submission to another require trust, unshakable trust. You have to dig even deeper to relinquish that trust to someone you cannot see. Yet God is very much alive. His faithfulness is beyond comprehension and His strength is unfailing. There is no one on this earth in Whom you can confide so confidently. I get so excited knowing God's love and faithfulness reaches so deeply into my heart. It careens into those secret places even I don't know exist. When I commit my life to Him, fully trusting His lead, I can feel secure knowing that any miracle He wants to perform in my life, He will perform.

Commitment means entrusting my life to God, with unwavering faith that He is in control. He knows what is best for me. He wants my life to shine for Him, and He will make it happen His way. When I earnestly seek to know Him better, He will disclose what He wants me to do, and how He wants me to do it. My responsibility is to continue to keep Him in His sacred place of honour in my life, reserving the throne of my heart only for Him.

What can I expect of Him? Miracles? Yes, miracles commissioned by the Master's touch. Some I am aware of, others I am not. Nevertheless, His miracles do take place according to His perfect plan. During the years immediately following my accident, I did not go through my journal entries. I needed to move forward with living and did not want to remain in the trauma of the past. One day, God wanted to "talk" to my heart. He wanted me to experience the reality of His faithfulness. As I reviewed some pages in my journals, God gently guided my heart to something specific.

The evening of the accident, Kip and I left home in separate vehicles. We were completely unaware of the trauma that would unfold only two kilometers from our home. God, on the other hand, had complete knowledge of every single detail. Within those few moments, He allowed certain things to happen. He also prevented certain things from happening. Why? I don't know, but He knew exactly what He would permit and what He would disallow. There were no surprises to Him and He was in complete control. Rereading this part of my journal, I felt as though He was tenderly providing some answers to my persistent questions of how to recognize miracles when they happen. Some were obvious, immediate and beyond question. Others, more subtle, required careful consideration and openness to God's leading. It also meant reliving a traumatic time, with my husband filling in the pieces I had not been aware of.

I began to recognize certain miracles that did take place that night. No one else had been severely hurt, and no passengers were in the van with me. Our precious family "pup" of nineteen years had passed away three days earlier. Had she been in the van, she likely would have been thrown through the windshield, as she loved to curl up on the front passenger seat. My husband, who had been following me in his own van, was protected from the collision. Our family physician had just come on duty when I arrived by ambulance at the hospital. And, I was alive!

Yes, God is opening my eyes. As I search His heart with sincere questions and a longing to draw closer in my understanding of Him, answers are gradually being revealed. I believe God knows when my heart is ready to decipher certain matters. Prior to this specified time, my heart was likely not able to grasp the significance of God's Divine Presence because of the initial effects of the accident. Perhaps I would not have acknowledged the abundance of miracles that did occur had I not desperately needed to seek God's comfort amid so much confusion. Others may view these occurrences as coincidence, but when one truly understands that the one and only God Almighty was, and is, in absolute control of the universe, there can be no doubt, *no* doubt whatsoever, that the Holy Spirit is an active participant in our lives.

Healing of the flesh is truly miraculous, and perhaps the most sought-after miracle. Healing of disease, illness and pain is generally accompanied by a positive, visual change within the body or mind. Jesus performed such miracles numerous times during His time on earth. Crowds followed Him hoping to simply touch His robe, hoping to receive His healing. However, during His lifetime on earth, Jesus was selective in His healing and He often decreed a proactive step of obedience and faith for the healing to take place. That act of obedience was the response of uninhibited faith. God does continue to physically heal. He may also call on fellow believers to lay their hands on one of His precious children, thus enabling His healing power to wash over them.

But there is another manner of divine healing that takes place which must not be overlooked. This type of healing is eternal and lasting. It does not depend on the temporary condition of the human body, which is always prone to disease, disability or infirmities. It does not fade as the body takes its normal course through the latter years of aging. Healing of the heart is of eternal importance, regardless of what takes place in the flesh. Paul reminds us of the frailty of our human bodies in 2 Corinthians 4:7–9, *"But we have this treasure in jars of clay to show that this all-surpassing power is from God, and not from us. We are hard pressed on every side, but not crushed; perplexed, but not in despair; persecuted, but not abandoned; struck down, but not destroyed."* Further down that passage he continues,

Therefore we do not lose heart. Though outwardly we are wasting away, yet inwardly we are being renewed day by day. For our light and momentary troubles are achieving for us an eternal glory that far outweighs them all. So we fix our eyes not on what is seen, but on what is unseen. For what is seen is temporary, but what is unseen is eternal. (2 Corinthians 4:16–18)

Realistically, my body is only a *temporary* vessel. It will fail me in one form or another. Our society digs its heels into the mud of resistance, desperate to slow down the aging process. We do everything we can to look and feel younger in a fruitless effort to remain younger. Caring for our bodies and living healthy lifestyles help us enjoy our lives much more fully, but it doesn't remove the reality that we are aging, and it doesn't guarantee freedom from illness, disability or death. Our bodies are temporal.

Without the Lord, I believe the journey would almost be unbearable to face, perhaps even rendering hopelessness. But God has created us to be spiritual human beings. We are not here simply to exist from birth to death. He has placed each one of us here to live, with purpose. We perish in fleshly body alone, our spirit being eternal and interminable. Knowing this truth transforms the apprehension of limited time on earth to anticipation of receiving eternal life! God dwells inside of me! He alone sits on the throne of my heart. Although my limitations may threaten to discourage me, and they do from time to time, I can still claim victory over them because I have Christ living inside of me. I am being spiritually renewed day by day! Access to Christ's divine power fulfills my life, enriching it daily as I walk with my hand in His, whether I am healthy, ill or disabled.

Reading further in 2 Corinthians, we find that Paul discloses battling a personal affliction which triggered health challenges. We do not know what the "thorn" was that Paul struggled with, but we do know that Paul must have been suffering substantially. He asked the Lord three times to remove it, but God did not. In 2 Corinthians 12:8–9, Paul states, *"Three times I pleaded with the Lord to take it away from me. But he said to me, 'My grace is sufficient for you, for my power is made perfect in weakness.'"*

Paul admits that he pleaded to have it removed. I'm sure, like most of us, Paul had times when he questioned why God chose not to remove it. He must have experienced bouts of frustration, as it is believed he was an active athlete. He was absolutely faithful to God, renouncing his formidable former way of life, and he rejoiced in a very personal relationship with the Lord God he grew to love so much. The Lord who filled him. The Lord who cleansed his heart. Yet at some point he experienced physical difficulties which God allowed to take place in his life. He wanted to move forward without them. He felt the thorn hindered the ministry he was called to do. But God replied that His grace was sufficient enough for Paul to do what God had called him to do. The Bible tells us of no further requests from Paul for the removal of his burden. Completely surrendered to the Lord God Almighty, his faith and trust remained unshakeable, and He accepted that God's strength would be seen instead of his own. Although his burden would remain, he trusted that God's grace would be sufficient.

God's promise to Paul was solid and powerful. It offered great hope to Paul that he was not alone, regardless of the barriers that seemed to mound up in front of him. God reminded Paul of His faithfulness and that His will would still be carried out regardless of the "thorn" Paul felt was a hindrance. Through God's grace, Paul was still used in a way that honoured and glorified God. He relied on God to show him how to be effective in his ministry, despite his limitations. This is a comforting fact for all of us when we recognize that Paul was a very strong and self-sufficient man. He was also an Apostle dedicating the remainder of his life to witnessing and professing the truth of God's Holy Word. Yet, God required humility from him. He also expected unbridled submission. Paul obeyed with a yielded heart and the power of God was magnified in his life.

Although God did not choose to remove this affliction from Paul, God did continue to perform miracles through Paul. The fact that God's grace was sufficient for Paul and God's power was made perfect through Paul's weakness, is a miracle in itself and cannot be ignored. Even today, Paul's relentless commitment to spread the Good News many centuries ago, despite his limitations, is continuing to bring millions to the gateway of eternal life through the life-saving message of the Lord Jesus Christ, the Messiah.

Paul grew to accept his limitations. He surrendered his weaknesses and his life to the God he grew to trust and love deeply. As a result, many others witnessed God's power at work. The Holy Bible records countless battles and struggles of physical restrictions experienced by those who loved the Lord God Almighty, yet all continued to trust Him, proclaiming His glory. Through their yielded hearts, God performed immeasurably profound miracles.

How many times has God performed miracles without our knowledge? I am a firm believer that God protects us from many harmful incidences. Some we are powerfully aware of, while others have produced no awareness whatsoever. Kip and I have seen His divine intervention many times. One trip in particular stimulated a distinct cognizance of His protection. Kip and I were finally able to slip away for one week of relaxation. We had planned to stay at one of our favourite lakes for three days, moving on from there to the city for the remainder of the week. Travelling to the city involved a much faster pace again, and there would be no quiet place to retreat to. However, we hadn't visited there for a long time.

On the last day at the lake, Kip asked if I would like to remain there for the entire holiday. We were really enjoying ourselves and the pace was light and very relaxing. Kip's suggestion underscored the time of renewal we were both benefiting from. The prospect of changing plans never occurred to me or Kip, until we started to prepare to leave. Embracing his suggestion, we decided to stay. Later that day, I wondered if God was protecting us from something. I do not usually get this feeling if or when we change plans; however, the feeling slipped in unannounced and was very strong at that moment. It then faded away as the afternoon progressed and I forgot about it.

The ensuing days were casual and very enjoyable. We could feel our bodies recharging as we walked, visited, and spent time on the lakeshore fishing. Kip enjoyed going to the clubhouse at the RV park every morning to socialize and have a cup of coffee. Friday morning, the television was on and there was quite a bit of discussion going on.

194

A murder had taken place at the very spot we would have been staying had we decided to continue on to our planned destination. Police had cordoned off the area, not allowing folks to come or go. Helicopters hovered above the area, while scuba divers searched the water below the docks, wharf and float houses. Total chaos enveloped the marina. We could not have escaped from it.

Immediately I thought of that one moment earlier in the week. I knew right then that God had gently spoken to our hearts, nudging us to remain where His peace would continue to strengthen us. How we praised the Lord for His protection! He knew we needed this time away and He knew the turmoil I would be in with so much activity, noise and confusion surrounding us with no way out until the police authorized us to leave. I wanted to hug the Lord so much as my heart soared with the realization of His protection and faithfulness. Reading again what the Dictionary says about the word miracle, I can attest to His wonders time and time again: "An extraordinary and welcome event believed to be the work of God…" I know God nudged us to stay put and on Friday the reason was revealed to us.

Awareness of this encourages me to remain vigilant, keeping my eyes and heart open to the unmistakable miracles God's given me and the blessing of knowing He will continue to do so. I deeply desire to be used by Him, and I want to declare the wonders He performs in my life, whether simple or grand! Sometimes external miracles of physical protection and physical healing are evident. Yet sometimes it is His choice not to intervene. However, there is no doubt in my heart that internal miracles of the yielded heart do take place with the promise of permanence, producing quality of life so profound we shout with joy, lifting our faithful God to His rightful place of honour. I want Him, and Him alone, on the throne of my heart.

I do not want to be blind to any miracle He has chosen to bless my life with, searching instead for other speculative miracles that would not produce the same fruit within me. I want to fix my eyes on what is unseen, because I am promised it is eternal.

I love Him immeasurably, and He promises to use me. Just as I am.

3

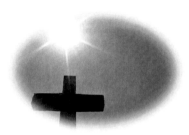

Encouragement and Support

Regardless of our standing in life, difficulties will always be present. Whether it is with our physical bodies, intellectual state of mind, struggles of the heart, or financial standing, every single human being encounters personal challenges at some point during the course of their lives. The severity and extent to which we struggle is individual and personal, but not one of us is exempt.

Words of encouragement are tiny little gems anyone can give away. Sincere and genuine kindness often lightens a heavy load from another's heart. True enough, the burden may remain, but words of encouragement and support can make an enormous difference in the loneliness often experienced during an extremely difficult time. The heartache of facing serious battles without the compassion and support of fellow believers in Christ can often trigger more pain than the difficult situation at hand.

To encourage means to uplift. As I contemplate this wonderful word, encouragement, many definitions swirl around endlessly in my head.

Words such as: build up, give confidence to, praise, inspire, cheer on, exhort, lift up, and reassure to name only a few. I have come to understand that these definitions translate through verbal acknowledgement: "Good job, great thinking, you did it, you've taken another step forward and I'm proud of you, you're doing really great." Genuine words of support and encouragement are a wonderful way to bring some sunshine into another person's life!

To cultivate the gift of encouragement, careful attention to what we say and how we say it is essential. Disheartening words must never be uttered. Words such as: "But if only, why can't you, but you used to, you've got to try harder, you're missing out, it's not all that bad, you'll get over it." These words are very discouraging to someone who has limitations, newly acquired or otherwise.

The Book of Proverbs is filled with verses revealing the significance of kindness, encouragement and support. Proverbs 12:25 is a wonderful example: *"An anxious heart weighs a man down, but a kind word cheers him up."* We all have discouraging times in our lives, but a kind word can initiate a smile. Receiving encouragement shines a little light into our life. Giving encouragement shines a little light into two lives, the life we are trying to make brighter, and our own life as we genuinely reach out with love. Life is rejuvenated when encouraging words fill an empty cup with hope. Proverbs 15:30 says, *"A cheerful look brings joy to the heart, and good news gives health to the bones."* An entire chapter could be written solely on individual verses found in Proverbs pertaining to the importance of encouragement, let alone within the rest of God's Word!

My husband Kip is my strongest anchor of encouragement, hands down. His incredible love, support and encouragement has led me to a place of complete security in who I am now. He has been my tireless motivator when I have felt defeated by failures. He has tuned into my spirit, drawing out the courage and determination he knows dwells inside of me. We have walked together hand in hand along this confusing pathway of change. He has reinforced his unshakeable love for me countless times, holding me when frustrations have flooded over me, bringing to the surface rivers of tears which had been swelling in the depths of my heart. He has tenderly wiped those tears away, steadfast with his genuine words of encouragement and support for each effort tackled, whether successful or not. He has also cried alongside of me at times, not only for the upheaval this disability has brought into our lives, but because he loves me so much that he *feels* the pain as though it were his.

My disability did not come with a handbook of instructions on what to expect, when to expect changes, or what things will work, nor explanations on how to avoid what won't work. There is absolutely no way to prepare myself for how to feel. Circumstances change daily. So does the choice to adapt, or fold under them. Each day is different and there is no recourse but to ceaselessly seek guidance, often groping my way as if in a mist or fog, not quite knowing what the answer is. Only through repetitive failure did I begin to recognize and face my newly acquired limitations. Early on, the effects of my disability quickly clarified the difference between "normal" then, and "normal" now. As the years pass, I have come to realize there are no gray or questionable areas with regard to certain functions. What is, now, always will be.

Unbelievable support, initially coming from my physician and highly respected brain injury specialists, made the road much less bumpy. I was commended for the adaptations I was making in my determination to find ways to live with this disability. In turn, support from professionals who didn't even know me enormously encouraged me to pursue the challenge of finding alternatives. As the disability and I became more familiar with each other, I began to look at the challenges differently. Instead of stepping back, afraid of failure, I progressively experienced an eagerness to conquer any limitation threatening to overpower me. I started to individualize challenges, reckoning each one as a challenge to overcome. This does not mean I always succeeded in my adaptations. I missed the mark many, many times. But through prayer, daily communion with my Lord, and recognition of my worth in His eyes, life took on new meaning. There was a focus, a goal, and a purpose once again.

1 Thessalonians chapter 5 presents countless ways to encourage a fellow human being. An encourager *builds up* another person, focusing on a special quality such as found even in the simplicity of a beautiful smile. An encourager is *patient, cheerful, ready to give assistance.* An

encourager speaks words of *genuine praise*. Words of discouragement, belittlement, ridicule, or doubt are never expressed. Affirming successes, regardless of how insignificant they may seem, sparks hope within the human soul. Genuine words of support and encouragement, especially from a loved one, can reignite awareness and acceptance of the power of the Holy Spirit's Fire, gradually restoring confidence and hope in the life of an individual.

Loyalty and commitment to go the distance with a friend or loved one significantly enriches the lives of all involved. Encouragement and unwavering support is articulated through various means, whether verbally spoken, written, physically or visually expressed, or even silently identified. It may be offered through those who love the Lord, or by those who don't know Him. However it is expressed, sincerity and authenticity through the act of encouragement can stabilize a heart's shaky foundation, generating renewed hope, trust and confidence. Authenticity and sincerity are the key elements of encouragement. Words void of truth and honesty are worthless, robbing not only the receiver but the giver as well.

Grateful for the encouragement and support that enriches my life, I am steadily growing stronger and more confident. My disability is no longer new to me, and I am learning to embrace the emergent familiarity. Doing so is gradually dispelling the aching desire inside to return to the life I used to have. Memory of life's former routine is becoming somewhat foggy as necessary adaptations have escorted me to the doorway of change. Successfully discovering those adaptations has greatly reduced my desire to look back. I am on a brand new path.

Life has become a lot more consistent, although I will admit the disability becomes very apparent when I am thrust into a situation which cannot be monitored. Such events or situations present uncertainty and internal trepidation as they represent unidentifiable bridges which I have not crossed before. During those times of particular vulnerability, I have often experienced enormous support, even from complete strangers whose help and compassion have certainly lessened the humility of embarrassment, especially when confusion makes me susceptible to dependency on someone else for safety reasons.

There are not always times of such reassurance. A Mild Traumatic Brain Injury is an invisible disability and its effects can set the stage for misunderstanding or misconstrued conceptions. A discouraging outcome can threaten to impede self-confidence and growth, and we cannot move forward in a healthy direction until *we* fully *accept ourselves.* Once we acquire an internal acceptance of who we are, the need to be accepted by others becomes secondary.

I have embraced the phrase, "Tomorrow has two handles: the handle of fear and the handle of faith. You can take hold of it by either handle" (Unknown). Surrendering this disability, which holds much unpredictability, to Almighty God was the changing point in my life. I didn't want to live in continual fear of the losses, physical and relational, which became more identifiable as time progressed.

I wanted life, abundant life! The only way to claim it was to surrender all of my fears to Him, to surrender my entire life to Him! Finally mustering up the courage to surrender everything to Him, I let go of the handle of fear and grasped tightly onto the handle of faith. "Let's go, Lord! I want to experience what you have in store for me!" I had to let go of who others thought I should be so I could focus solely on the pathway God was guiding me to. I was doing everything in my own human power to move forward, but to reduce uncertainty it was crucial to fix my eyes on Jesus without glancing sideways or backward.

Through His grace, God has enlightened my understanding. The dearest of friends and loved ones have celebrated my achievements and remained loyal through failures. Their encouragement has often prompted me to take the risk to try again, but with a different approach. They pick me up, dust me off, give me a hug then set me free to walk with assurance along the pathway God has placed me on. They focus on the strengths and gifts I still possess, spurring me on to discover how to use those blessings. Loving and gentle reminders have enabled me to recognize and accept new boundaries now in place. They encourage me as I step forward, but never once shove me to go faster, farther or beyond the capabilities I now possess. They rejoice with me in little *and* big successes.

New friendships have budded since the accident, but they have had a little easier introduction to my disability. They never knew me prior to the accident, so acceptance of who I am has flourished, our friendships deepening as they are cultivated on both sides. This is also the case for little children. There is nothing to compare me to. I'm just me. They don't look for more than what I can be, because in their innocence, "what is" is good enough. There is no awareness of a disability. It is very freeing, for all of us.

Some have educated themselves on the effects of my disability, either through research on the Internet, reading books or material describing brain injury and its effects, or through other relevant resources. They genuinely want to learn more because they love enough to care. This in turn helps them understand why I need to say no to certain things, what triggers confusion and fatigue, how to recognize certain signals, and why it is important to stay within my boundaries.

I love them so very much for the importance and value they place on the relationship between us. Their unpretentious efforts to accept me just as I am, without pressure to be someone I can no longer be, enable me to progress more confidently. There is no advantage in looking backward, as that is when we trip and fall the hardest. Unbiased acceptance, encouragement and support from these friends and loved ones have led me to experiment and engage in new activities, exposing gifts longing to be unwrapped. As a result I am able to be free, just to be me!

The example of these faithful human treasures in my life triggers a passionate desire to do the same for others. I want to be used by God and I know He wants to use me. Encouragement is a gem not only to be received but also given away. I do have the ability to encourage at least one person *every single day*, whether verbally, through an email, or perhaps by way of a handwritten note. The gift of encouragement must be genuine. Seeking to encourage someone else lifts my eyes off myself and my inadequacies, and grants me the privilege to acknowledge another in a positive way.

My eyes and heart are now wide open to the message God is giving me. Although I am at home most days of the week, I am still able to encourage others, filling my days with a healthy and unselfish focus. There is such tremendous value in placing others above yourself. This outward focus has brought an affluence of contentment into my life. God has great work for me to do, and I overflow with excitement when I consider the endless possibilities!

Faithfulness and genuine encouragement, particularly through rough times, can produce a spark of hope amidst present darkness. A word, a touch, a note, an affirmation, a smile, a hug, a prayer, a shoulder (or perhaps even a bucket), are all indicative signs of an encourager. Scripture identified a fellow named Barnabas as an encourager. His real name was Joseph. Acts 4:36 explains: *"The apostles called [him] Barnabas (which means Son of Encouragement)."* Acts 11:23–24 elaborates: *"When he arrived and saw the evidence of the grace of God, he was glad and encouraged them all to remain true to the Lord with all their hearts. He was a good man, full of the Holy Spirit and faith, and a great number of people were brought to the Lord."* This fellow was definitely an encourager! First, he recognized the grace of God. Expounding on that, he found the positive in situations, and he encouraged others to do the same.

The act of encouragement is addressed several times within God's Holy Word. It is not limited to the healthy, wealthy, wise or religious. It is a gift we can all share to build up another human being, particularly during hard times. Matthew 5:14–16 says,

> *You are the light of the world. A city on a hill cannot be hidden. Neither do people light a lamp and put it under a bowl. Instead they put it on its stand, and it gives light to everyone in the house. In the same way, let your light shine before men, that they may see your good deeds and praise your Father in heaven.*

I am a very visual person. Reading this passage produces a virtual video inside of my head. I visualize a bright lamp being put under a bowl, darkness instantly blanketing the room. Fear and uncertainty can be powerful forces when there is darkness. Next, I see the lamp placed on a table, not only filling the room with light but also producing a sense of comfort. Light gives us vision to see, helping us determine all that is around us.

I want to radiate faithfulness and compassion so others can experience the love of God! I want to be that lamp, exposing God's love for them. I want to be a source of encouragement, used by God to blanket someone else with comfort and support as they endure suffering. I want to feel the hurt when someone else is hurting, because I personally know how comforting it is to be held in loving arms which silently say, "I'm here for you." On the flipside, I want to share the joy of someone who is celebrating. It is exhilarating to hear someone bubble over with excitement because something special has brightened their life!

When God nudges me to write to someone, I will write. When He nudges me to send a pretty flower to brighten someone's day, I will call the florist. Perhaps a simple homemade gift would bring a smile, "just because." Even an email can offer an invitation for someone to come over when they are hurting, to be held or to openly weep in the security of a trusted friendship. An outward focus is mandatory in order for endless opportunities to surface every day.

No one lights a lamp only to put it under a bowl. The result would be encompassing darkness. Instead, they put it on its stand where it gives light and comfort to everyone in its presence. That's how it is with the gift of encouragement and support. Radiating God's love through unselfish gifts of encouragement and support lightens not only the hearts of those we expose it to, it warmly reflects back to our own hearts, filling us with joy and completeness in who we are in Jesus Christ!

4

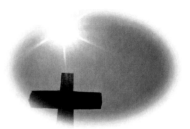

HOPE

"We wait in hope for the LORD; he is our help and our shield. In him our hearts rejoice, for we trust in his holy name. May your unfailing love rest upon us, O LORD, even as we put our hope in you." (Psalm 33:20–22)

Timeless, eternal hope swells inside my very being as I grip tightly to the hand of the One Who controls my future. Any threat of gloom is dispelled when I call upon His name. God, the Eternal One, is in control of our very lives, asking only that we trust Him entirely with each and every aspect of our humanness. Sometimes that seems hard to comprehend. In my humanness I cannot see past certain moments or certain situations, but God can. His mighty power has proved faithful in miraculous ways since the beginning of time.

Paul discusses the hope of eternal glory, accessible to all God's children through the salvation we receive the instant we accept Jesus Christ as our Lord and Saviour. Paul says in Romans 8:24–28,

For in this hope we were saved. But hope that is seen is no hope at all. Who hopes for what he already has? But if we hope for what we do not yet have, we wait for it patiently. In the same way, the Spirit helps us in our weakness. We do not know what we ought to pray for, but the Spirit himself intercedes for us with groans that words cannot express. And he who searches our hearts knows the mind of the Spirit, because the Spirit intercedes for the saints in accordance with God's will. And we know that in all things God works for the good of those who love him, who have been called according to his purpose.

What incredible promises! Take some time to read it through again. Break it down. *Write* it down and put your name into it. Digest it. Absorb it. Close all else out of your mind and commune with God. *You* are His child. Let His truth give you understanding of the powerful message contained within these verses. This passage offers immense comfort and endless hope to those who are seeking His will.

Words are often elusive when we face suffering or tragedy and we don't understand what is happening or why. Tears may flow or we may feel numb inside. God searches our hearts and the Holy Spirit intercedes on our behalf when words just won't come! That's how incredibly personal God is with His children! He doesn't say, "Well, when you remember what you wanted to tell me, come back and try again." Nor does He say, "When you can collect yourself enough so I can understand you, *then* come back and talk to me." No, instead He feels our agony and pain and He recognizes that even words cannot be defined to express what's in our hearts sometimes. Searching between and through the crevices of our inner being, He shines His light of compassion on the source of pain. Exposing the source, He is then ready to work through it with us, giving rise to the hope which is accessible to all who call Him Father.

Paul encourages us to remember that hope which is seen is really no hope at all. Why would we lay issues before Christ if we already knew what lay ahead? If we already knew the outcome? Paul wants us to understand that if the storybook of our lives was revealed to us from beginning to end, there would be no hope for the future. The outcome would be ascertained and our days would become mediocre. We would exist but without choices, rendering our lives stagnant. We would die, without having had any purpose.

Paul asks a pertinent question, *"Who hopes for what he already has?"* Our bodies are temporary but our souls are eternal. The hope we have for everlasting life comes only through the blood of our Lord Jesus Christ. What lies ahead of us is only known to our Creator, Who is Almighty God. I don't want to know what lies ahead, although I will concede having wondered during various stages of difficulty how on earth everything would turn out. I'm sure we have all experienced those feelings at one time or another. Yet that's what makes hope in Jesus Christ so profound! As a child of God, I can surrender the outcome to the One Who has ordained all of my days!

One day, I had the enormous pleasure of enjoying a visit with a lovely young woman. During our conversation, she mentioned taking a trip to see her grandfather. Her heart ached to see his body so physically disabled, dependent on others for care. She wondered why God would choose to let our bodies break down the way they often do as we age. I believe her honest question is asked by hundreds of thousands of people all over the world. I thought about her question a lot that evening. It is not only the aging process that causes our bodies to break down. Many other factors can take place in the human life, causing physical weakness, disability or ill-health, regardless of age. However, for her at this point and time, the question was focused on her grandfather whom she loves so much.

I pondered the passage in 2 Corinthians 4:16–18 which offers some guidance to that question: *"Therefore we do not lose heart. Though outwardly we are wasting away, yet inwardly we are being renewed day by day. For our light and momentary troubles are achieving for us an **eternal** glory that far outweighs them all. So we fix our eyes not on what is seen, but on what is unseen. For what is seen is temporary, but what is unseen is eternal"* (emphasis mine).

I sat down and wrote her a note, passing on these verses. She is a strong Christian and undoubtedly knows this passage; however, I wanted to encourage her to embrace God's faithfulness by continuing on through 2 Corinthians 5:1–10, which describes God's promises of an eternal heavenly home, *"not built by human hands"* (2 Corinthians 5:2). Paul talks about the frailty of the human body and how we, as Christians, should not get too comfortable in our fleshly *"tents."* As we've read previously, Paul personally experienced how frail our earthly bodies can be. He encourages us to focus on pleasing God daily by surrendering our will to His.

It's important not to depend on the physical strengths of our humanness, as they are temporary and fleeting. God wants us to be restless about permanency while we exist on this earth. He wants us to always look ahead to the Kingdom He has prepared for us. Yet it is critical to remember that it is only in His perfect timing that we will be transported to our eternal Home with Him. Until He calls us Home, there is still work to be done whether we recognize it or not. What is significant is that God continues to work in us even through the frailty of our earthly bodies. He will often work in ways we may not recognize or understand, but we must remember that He is in control at all times, in each and every life He has created. Our promise from Him affirms that when our work on earth is finished, He will bring us Home to eternal glory.

My mother is in her eighties. She is blind in one eye and can barely see out of the other. She has broken her ankle, shoulder, and wrist, and cracked her pelvis. She has osteoporosis and she is getting hard of hearing. These are the ailments I can *remember!* My mother has always been heavily involved in God's work, her focus fixed on witnessing for her Lord. She has co-written a prayer book sent out by her home church, finding its way all around the world. Spanning many decades, my mother has written and addressed hundreds of devotions for various church groups. She has provided lunch on Sundays in her apartment for guests who are young, middle-aged, or elderly. Age does not matter. She is a true prayer warrior, lifting many up in prayer, including her daughter. She has visited those in hospital or care facilities for countless years. Her entire life has been driven by the passionate desire to serve others in Christ's name.

Conquering the task of emailing, through the patient training of my brother, she fills her "letters" with the week's events and ends up "running off the page," as "there is not enough room!" My brother has since taught her how to scroll down, so the "letters" continue to grow! How she does this with her partial and dim eyesight is beyond comprehension.

The subject line on one of her latest emails read, "GOD STILL HAS WORK FOR ME TO DO!" She went on to explain that she has been asked to take part in redesigning an invitation for first-time guests in her church wishing to have a visit from one of the church ministry staff. Then she wrote something I have set apart to remind me of the hope and joy experienced when serving Christ, regardless of what life has led us through. She wrote, "Remember what I said at my (80th) birthday party? I want to serve Him as long as He gives me breath. I am so happy He is providing opportunities! I think that is why He gave me this "Blessing" so I could fulfill what I testified to do, with God's grace!" (The word "Blessing" is a reference to the computer she received upon the passing of a dear friend.)

My mother ended her email with this last comment, "I sure get carried away on this 'Blessing' and before I know it I have written a book!!" Like mother, like daughter. We both love Jesus so much, and we both depend on Him for the deepest kind of joy imaginable. She has been through so many heart-wrenching trials in her lifetime, yet she continues to fix her eyes upon Jesus. Her heart's door is swung wide open to His leading, and for her, there is no other option. He has proven His faithfulness to her time and time again, and I have had the privilege of being witness to the impact He has made in her life.

There is no greater joy for my mother on this earth than to serve others as if she were literally serving Him. She is aging. She is not free of pain, but she *is* free! Her body fails her at times, but her Lord does not. He never has. He is the eternal beacon of hope she turns to, and He has carried her faithfully through numerous valleys of struggles and heartache, instilling in her an eternal awareness of the word hope.

Her hunger for Him has whetted my spiritual appetite. She has walked through the phases of my brain injury since she first learned of the accident. She has guided me, cried with me, encouraged me, grounded me and ceaselessly prayed for me. She has also done the same for Kip, recognizing the changes it has brought to his life, and to our life together. But more than all of this, she has tirelessly yet gently reminded me, and us, of the hope that is realized through our Lord and Saviour Jesus Christ. He is the anchor we must always hold onto.

Her words are never harsh, accusing, belittling or testing. She is an encourager and her words build up, never tear down. She radiates compassion and wisdom, encouraging us as a couple to fix our eyes only on Jesus for guidance, direction and strength. I am her daughter, but I belong to God. She often reminds me that she can advise, however I must fix my eyes on Jesus and ultimately seek His direction. These are truths she wants me to personally experience in my intimate walk with the Saviour. He is the Hope Eternal, the *only* Hope Eternal. Dependence upon anyone or anything else is unhealthy and will only lead to disappointment, endless discouragement and emptiness.

I have made choices and decisions that have been wrong. Innocent and thoughtless mistakes surface much quicker than I want them to, and they will continue to do so. That's what makes me human, and sinful. However, I am responsible to seek forgiveness from God and from whomever I may hurt, innocently or otherwise, making every effort possible not to repeat those mistakes, but to learn from them. I want to grow wiser, deepening my walk with God, and I do not want to stunt my growth by being a repeat offender with no regard for the lessons needing to be learned. God has given me life and I don't want to waste or misuse any element of it!

By contrast, my Heavenly Father is divine, pure and completely sinless. He is the reason there is forgiveness. His Omnipotence enables me to place complete, unwavering trust and hope in Who He is, the only One Who can do what I cannot. The freedom available through His Son Jesus Christ to each and every human being offers immense and eternal hope which reaches far beyond ourselves to an entire world that suffers from immeasurable emotional and physical pain.

God is the Creator, of everything. He speaks and the earth trembles. His very words formed the earth with all of its majesty as He carefully fashioned every intricate detail. How then can I ever doubt His tender care and concern in every aspect of my life? Indubitably, I have doubted sometimes. Ecclesiastes 3:11–12 says, *"He has made everything beautiful in its time. He has also set eternity in the hearts of men; yet they cannot fathom what God has done from beginning to end. I know that there is nothing better for men than to be happy and do good while they live."*

When the apple cart of life tips over, spilling uncertainty onto the road we are travelling, doubt can encompass our thoughts because it is a more tangible feeling to give in to. At times, we have an acute awareness of the problems, limitations, and difficulties facing us. Enshrouded by the fog of doubt, we are not able to see a brighter tomorrow or lasting solutions. The victorious truth is that God has full knowledge of what lies past that upset apple cart. Should we choose to allow Him to guide us through the tragedy, the mess, the helplessness, we will discover beautiful and eternal treasures waiting just beyond the last bruised apple lying on the ground.

Another of my cherished Bible verses is found in Philippians 4:4–8:

Rejoice in the Lord always. I will say it again: Rejoice! Let your gentleness be evident to all. The Lord is near. Do not be anxious about anything, but in everything by prayer and petition, with thanksgiving, present your requests to God. And the peace of God, **which transcends all understanding,** *will guard your hearts and your minds in Christ Jesus. Finally, brothers, whatever is* **true,** *whatever is* **noble,** *whatever is* **right,** *whatever is* **pure,** *whatever is* **lovely,** *whatever is* **admirable**—*if anything is excellent or praiseworthy—think about such things.* (Emphasis mine)

First I am instructed to praise Him regardless how difficult things may be. Upon doing this, there stands a rich promise that God's peace will flood over my soul, surpassing my human comprehension. It will guard my heart and mind from doubt, fear, uncertainty, apprehension and hopelessness because my trust rests in the Lord Jesus. Next, the Lord promises to be near. That guarantees He is with me every second of every day. Subsequently, I am instructed not to be anxious, about anything! He tells me to bring everything before Him, with thanksgiving! Lastly, I am commanded to think about truth, dignity, graciousness, fairness, purity, loveliness, admiration and excellence.

Constant focus on these virtues will make it exceptionally difficult for Satan to access any part of my mind or heart. His sole motivation is to rob my life of the joy and purpose laid out for me through God's plan. God did not create a puppet to manipulate; He gives me freedom to make choices. I can choose to cower with Satan, shrinking beneath the load, choosing hopelessness by continuing to recoil when faced with limitations, challenging circumstances, disappointments and failures. I can grumble and complain about the rotten hand that has been dealt me. In contrast, I can stand tall in spirit, shoulders back, head held high, eyes fixed forward to embrace the rich eternal hope offered freely to me through my Lord and Saviour, Jesus Christ. As it is for my mother, it is for me; however, my faith does not exist because it is my mother's faith. My faith exists because I've personally experienced God's Presence, His faithfulness and His power all through my childhood years, then beyond, to where I am today.

There is no option for me but to freely live within God's purpose for my life. I choose to stand humbled, yet tall in spirit, secure in knowing God's grace will lead me to abundant living because of the hope I have in Him and through Him. As I place unrelenting faith in the divine Trinity of Father, Son and Holy Spirit, the vision beyond the hills and mountains of challenge is illuminated with the priceless treasure of immeasurable hope.

"Let us hold unswervingly to the hope we profess, for he who promised is faithful." (Hebrews 10:23)

5

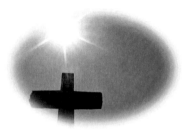

Worthy!

Through intense soul searching over the past several years, there is one constant that remains concrete and everlasting. My life is of eternal worth in my Father's eyes. I am worthy to be part of His awe-inspiring creation, worthy of His enduring and unconditional love, worthy of His salvation, and worthy to be His child. Nothing in my life has changed, nor ever could change, the ultimate purpose for which He intended when He intricately created me.

Fullness of this understanding took me years to comprehend and will take the rest of my life to continually bear in mind. I could identify with it more easily when life was coasting along comfortably, however it was much more difficult to grasp when my brain injury occurred, particularly through the early phases of identification. The battle with Satan is not done until I am Home with my Lord. It is a very serious battle, one in which my spiritual armour will protect me as long as I take the responsibility of "suiting up" properly. Complete instructions for placement are clearly found in God's Holy Word (Ephesians 6:10–18).

I only want to walk upon the path God has chosen for me. The directions may not always be clear, but God promises to lead me and I willingly surrender to His guidance. I will glance sideways, trip, fall, weep and "fail" many times, yet every time God's unconditional love will reach down to help me up. He will rescue me from despair and He will strengthen my heart and my spirit. He has done so in the past and He will continue to do so as long as I live on this earth.

David experienced similar emotions. He says in Psalm 103:8–13,

The LORD is compassionate and gracious, slow to anger, abounding in love. He will not always accuse, nor will he harbour his anger forever; he does not treat us as our sins deserve or repay us according to our iniquities. For as high as the heavens are above the earth, so great is his love for those who fear him; as far as the east is from the west, so far has he removed our transgressions from us. As a father has compassion on his children, so the LORD has compassion on those who fear him.

Providing my heart is sincere in my walk with Him, I can rest secure in knowing He will be tirelessly patient with me and He will wisely guide and instruct me. His love is so vast it cannot be contained. His Holy Word affirms that each life is worth that kind of insurmountable, unconditional love!

God has not placed a "conditions" sticker on my life that reads, "This life will lose its value if scratched, broken, disfigured or damaged in any way, rendering it worthless." Circumstances, often beyond our control, do scratch, damage and break us emotionally, physically and spiritually. In the book of 1 Samuel, the Lord spoke to Samuel, clearly indicating what He considers to be of great worth in a person, *"But the LORD said to Samuel, 'Do not consider his appearance or his height, for I have rejected him. The LORD does not look at the things man looks at. Man looks at the outward appearance, but the LORD looks at the heart'"* (1 Samuel 16:7). Although the man before Samuel had a pleasing and impressive outward appearance, God made it very clear that the qualities Samuel visually admired were not the qualities God sought after.

God sees no disability. He does not turn away or remain distant because I am "different." In fact, He sees me the way He has always seen me, as His creation. Acts 17:28 says, *"For in him we live and move and have our being.' As some of your own poets have said, 'We are his offspring.'"* Amazing, isn't it? God loves us so incredibly much that we who believe upon His name are heirs to His Kingdom, His Eternal Home, His Mansion of Glory! Romans 8:16–17 promises, *"The Spirit himself testifies with our spirit that we are God's children. Now if we are children, then we are heirs—heirs of God and co-heirs with Christ, if indeed we share in his sufferings in order that we may also share in his glory."* My "suffering" seems so insignificant when contrasted with my Saviour's suffering during His short time on this earth. Yet my suffering has been experienced by my Saviour.

To live for Jesus is to renounce certain practices acceptable in the world's eyes but not acceptable to God. To live for Jesus requires a commitment to make Him the one and only God I will worship. This commitment is not always accepted or understood, and standing on solid ground in my walk with Him can, and does, bring about suffering. But I cannot do otherwise, because I love Him so much. In my mind there is no "Options" button to click. I can personally attest to His faithfulness—above anything else I trust Him implicitly.

What a powerful promise this passage concludes with: *"...that we may also share in his glory."* Wow, I am God's kid! I automatically became an heir to His Eternal Kingdom the moment I accepted Jesus Christ as my personal Saviour. I committed to follow His leading and to live as He asks. I have not abandoned that commitment because I now have a disability. I realize there will times of wavering, and of failure, but as long as I genuinely endeavor to do God's will, remaining committed to my new life in Him, eternal life with Jesus is guaranteed! The Bible verifies that eternity is not spent "somewhere," thank goodness! Rather, we are promised an eternal inheritance in which we shall be united with the One Who created us. We have been chosen and are worthy to live in God's Kingdom! His Kingdom, forever! It's almost too much for our finite human minds to comprehend. But it is promised to us!

Romans 8:28 encourages, *"And we know that in all things God works for the good of those who love him, who have been called according to his purpose."* I do love Him ever so much! I can have unwavering confidence that God will work everything in my life for good as He desires to fulfill His purpose for my life. I may not always feel everything is working out for the good, but that's where I must surrender and trust God to fulfill His promise. That gives my life not only earthly value and worth, but eternal value and worth as well! Isaiah 43:1 says, *"Fear not, for I have redeemed you; I have summoned you by name; you are mine.'"* By name! Excitement rushes through me as I cherish these promises from God, my Heavenly Father!

I am God's masterpiece. This is not a conceited thought; it is a divine affirmation of God's intricate design of His creation. Me, as well as you! Ephesians 2:10 says, *"For we are God's workmanship, created in Christ Jesus to do good works, which God prepared in advance for us to do."* This Scripture reminds me that my life has significant worth and enormous value as God's child. To feel inferior or less of a person, with or without a disability, would be an insult to God, the Creator of my life. He has specifically prepared work for me to do and it is my responsibility as His child to make the most of His workmanship!

God is indifferent to my disability. He sees me as His child who needs direction, guidance and love. I must depend on Him to show me what He expects of me, and then I must move forward to accomplish His purpose. Ephesians 5:8–10 says, *"Live as children of light (for the fruit of the light consists in all goodness, righteousness and truth) and find out what pleases the Lord."* To reflect Jesus, I need to have confidence in who I am. I need to recognize my worth in Christ; it is crucial to serving others. Respect for who I am, exactly as I am, radiates Christ's life in mine. I want others to see Him, to know Him and to fully experience their priceless worth in Him.

It has taken time to untangle the broken and damaged roots of my self-worth since the accident. I have struggled a great deal with feelings of sadness, frustration, timidity, guilt, doubt and loneliness. Not wanting to succumb to the fruitless place of helplessness and self-pity, I knew I needed to search for understanding of what God wanted for my life. Reviewing personal journals, I recognize more clearly now how those times of painful emotions and struggles inaugurated personal and spiritual growth. Years of self-evaluation deepened my relationship with the Heavenly Father and rekindled self-renewal, enabling me to experience true joy once again.

1 Thessalonians 5:16–19 says, *"Be joyful always; pray continually; give thanks in all circumstances, for this is God's will for you in Christ Jesus. Do not put out the Spirit's fire."* I get immensely excited about the Spirit's Fire! This passage is powerful! Utilizing the gifts God has blessed me with makes my life radiate with the Spirit's Fire, freely allowing the Holy Spirit to work through me. Enormous joy encompasses my soul as I embrace those words, initiating optimistic anticipation of the discovery of new blessings! Through relinquishing my uncertainties, I am wholeheartedly able to receive the power of the Holy Spirit. God loves me so much He divinely made provision for the Holy Spirit to dwell within me. This divine provision is available to all who believe upon His name.

Opening my heart's door to Christ not only invites Him to sit on the throne of my heart, it also denies Satan, the father of lies, access to any part of my being. God Almighty promises to be present in each and every circumstance I encounter. He promises to be there in the heat of trials, daily challenges and unwelcome struggles. He also promises to be there for continuous self-renewal discovered only through personal victory. Yet there is an even greater promise God gives—His promise for Eternal life. When I put my trust and faith in the resurrection of the Risen Saviour, declaring Him Lord of my life, He promises the assurance of eternal life with Him. John 3:16 says, *"For God so loved the world that he gave his one and only Son, that whoever believes in him shall not perish but have eternal life."* Looking beyond this earthly, temporary shell of flesh and bone, I firmly hold onto the promise of my Lord that my body will no longer have limitations; my disability will not exist.

I am familiar with the harsh reality of disabilities. Long before my accident, I was witness to an extremely severe disability in a young boy who was the son of a dear friend. The Lord took him Home at the age of ten. Following that Christ-honouring funeral, I sobbed without shame as I listened to that glorious song, *In the Garden*. In its entirety, this song reassures believers of the solid guarantee we have for eternal life with Jesus beyond these "jars of clay."

The following words in particular washed over me, saturating my heart with unfathomable love and gratitude for what I lay claim to as God's chosen child: "And, He walks with me and He talks with me, and *He tells me I am His own.* And the joy we share as we tarry there, none other has ever known" (emphasis mine). This family experienced great heartache and anguish, but they also loved Jesus! They trusted Him implicitly through challenges, difficulties, and endless trials, yet woven between the threads of despair was an internal peace that could only come from complete dependence on God Almighty.

As the words flooded my soul that day I knew, *really knew,* this young boy was now complete in his fullness. I pictured him walking with Jesus, side by side, experiencing one-on-one conversation with Him, experiencing the joy of being whole for all of eternity! None of us truly knows what Heaven will be like, but we do know God has promised each one of His children that it will be more breathtaking than we could ever humanly envision. That beautiful, picturesque song fills my heart with incredible hope and anticipation of how glorious eternity with Him will be.

This young boy's time on earth was not a mistake. God knew exactly what He was doing with His creation. Many lives were touched by the witness of his Christ-honouring parents, who loved him ever so much. It was a very difficult load to bear. There were other young lives to nurture and care for, and I cannot truly know the fullness of how it tested every aspect of their lives. But this young boy was their precious child. He was also God's precious child. Although his extreme disability prevented him from actively participating in life, his very being was of incredible worth to the Lord God Almighty. When Christ received him Home, he entered into eternity as an heir to the Kingdom of the One Who created him. His parents *will* see him again, in the divine wholeness promised to each and every believer.

Revelation 21:4 says, *"He will wipe every tear from their eyes. There will be no more death or mourning or crying or pain, for the old order of things has passed away."* What comforting promises! To try to grasp the full meaning of that verse would be futile, for we are only human and know only human realities. Yet that is what faith is all about. Believing, knowing and trusting in that which you cannot rationalize.

Christ loves me so much that He was willing to die on the cross so I could share eternity with Him! It is an honour to lift Him up as Lord, confidently depending on Him daily as I strive to do His will. Placing my focus on Christ and the sacrifice of His life for mine, acknowledging that God loves me to that extent, enables me to truly experience the value of my life in God's eyes. John 1:12 says, *"Yet to all who **received** him, to those who **believed in his name,** he gave the **right** to become **children of God**"* (emphasis mine). What He did for me, and you, validates our worthiness! Regardless of what takes place in our lives, nothing can compare with God's infinite compassion, unconditional love, and ultimate forgiveness. 1 John 3:1 says, *"How great is the love the Father has lavished on us, that we should be called children of God!"*

It is important to have a healthy understanding of the spiritual balance which must take place in order to correctly understand our worth in Christ. Yes, we are worthy simply because we are God's children. But the greatest understanding of our worthiness can only be found through the blood of Jesus. Sinless, He bore each individual's sin upon His shoulders, declaring victory over death through His resurrection three days later, so all could inherit eternal life. His blood was shed for us, in place of ours. Through this sacrifice we are empowered to have direct access to God the Father, through the blood of Jesus Christ, His Son.

Our relationship with Almighty God, along with our eternal inheritance, depends not on what we are able to do, nor does it depend on who we are in the world's standing. There is no legalistic ladder of good deeds upon which to climb toward Heaven. What if there were? How far could we climb before humanly falling as a result of sin? Would we have to start all over again and, if so, would we ever be able to succeed? What if our interpretation of "good deeds" and moral ethics is different than God's? What if His list of rules is humanly unattainable? How could we enjoy abundant life without being obsessively worried about falling off the rungs? How could we share His love with others when we need to constantly focus on how we are going to reach the top ourselves? Would we step on top of others to get there first? Would we think so highly of ourselves during our successes that our hearts would become blind to the needs of others? Could we live with ourselves should we slip or fall, failure loudly mocking from the legalistic ladder above?

Praise God this isn't the way to Heaven! Not one human being on this earth would ever be able to climb that impossible and hopeless ladder! There is no point system. If there were, Heaven would be unattainable! The way to Heaven is simple, and trustworthy. The only way to Heaven is by accepting Jesus Christ as Lord and Saviour of our lives, entering into a personal relationship with Him. John 14:6 defines this clearly, *"Jesus answered, 'I am the way and the truth and the life. No one comes to the Father except through me."* Prior to this passage spoken by Jesus is another clarification of what it means to have a personal relationship with Him. In John 10:27–30, Jesus says, *"My sheep listen to my voice; I know them, and they follow me. I give them eternal life, and they shall never perish; no one can snatch them out of my hand. My Father, who has given them to me, is greater than all; no one can snatch them out of my Father's hand. I and the Father are one."*

The Christian faith is a faith that stands all on its own. There is no legalistic ladder to climb and there are no step-by-step procedures that must be followed in order to reach God. There is no statue or manmade image that can determine your spiritual future. Recently, a preacher I respect a great deal shared the simplicity of the Christian faith with his congregation. The simplistic truth of the Christian faith is discovered in the understanding that God reaches down to us, His children. He meets us where we are at. If we fall, He gently picks us up. If we sin, then genuinely confess and repent of that sin, He readily forgives. In fact, we become justified through the blood of Jesus. Complete freedom is attained within the heart of a repentant believer. More than forgiven, justification declares that the sin itself is no longer remembered by our Lord. The slate is clear and untarnished. Can you grasp the enormity of how much your life is worth? God alone is perfect and He has done what no other can to declare His incredible love for you!

In John 14:15–21 Jesus says,

If you love me, you will obey what I command. And I will ask the Father, and he will give you another Counsellor to be with you forever—the Spirit of truth. The world cannot accept him, because it neither sees him nor knows him. But you know him, for he lives with you and will be in you. I will not leave you as orphans; I will come to you. Before long, the world will not see me anymore, but you will see me. Because I live, you also will live. On that day you will realize that I am in my Father, and you are in me, and I am in you. Whoever has my commands and obeys them, he is the one who loves me. He who loves me will be loved by my Father, and I too will love him and show myself to him.

Read that passage again and really study it. We are not orphans; rather we are heirs to the eternal Kingdom of God. The plan and purpose for my life and yours has been designed so intricately there can be no doubt of our immense worth to God Almighty.

I am His child! I am worthy in His eyes, and so are you!

APPENDIX

WHAT IS ACQUIRED BRAIN INJURY?

THE ANGELS WERE PRESENT NOVEMBER 7, 2001. THAT I KNOW. GOD didn't give them instructions to stop the car accident, nor did He give them instructions to bring me Home. Instead, He allowed my life to be extremely altered, and I had to face a new direction in my journey. Uncertainty, frustration, confusion, and pain were the first stepping stones at the base of the new mountain I was challenged to climb.

Outwardly, there were no obvious signs of physical impairment, yet internal damage to my brain produced an invisible disability forcing me into a world of unfamiliarity. I was also not alone. My "normal" world as of November 6, 2001, was encircled with many loved ones, personal friends and respected business associates. Like the rippling effect of a stone thrown into the water, the results and challenges of this newly acquired disability touched everyone involved in my life. Suddenly, life itself became very unpredictable.

Years of education, counselling and medical support enabled me to cross the bridge of uncertainty, strengthening each step through awareness. Reaching for God's hand and finding it already outstretched empowered me to grow *beyond* awareness to a place of spiritual fulfillment and contentment with who I am, in His eyes.

Millions of people suffer from acquired traumatic brain injuries, the intruder often remaining nameless because it is invisible. Silently, they battle this unseen adversary, not wanting to be "different," yet life keeps getting harder to cope with. I was extremely fortunate to have a very astute physician who probed for answers.

The following information was provided by the Powell River Brain Injury Society, a strong support group for those suffering from acquired brain injuries. It is an excellent summary of what defines an acquired brain injury, what produces an acquired brain injury, and indicative symptoms of a brain-injured person. Awareness is increasing, however there is a long way to go.

Perhaps you have witnessed someone at the check-out in front of you who seems to be terribly slow, and you are in a rush. Take into consideration that cognitive challenges may be the culprit. Perhaps a young person (without a helmet) took a bad tumble on their bicycle, and days later is uncharacteristically struggling to accomplish their school work. Have that bump on the head checked over more carefully. Maybe someone you love was involved in a car accident, walking away with only bumps and bruises, yet they have begun to exhibit signs of confusion, frustration and memory problems. Be patient with them, and seek further medical investigation.

Whether *enabled* or *disabled,* I encourage each reader to give the widest berth of consideration and compassion to everyone they interact with. We all have good days along with bad days, successes and failures, strengths and weaknesses. Strive to genuinely uplift and encourage at least one person every day, whether you feel like it or not. The gift of encouragement will not only lighten someone else's day, it will also lighten yours. Radiate Christ's love and *your* life will shine. And every morning, look in the mirror with confidence, secure in the assurance that **you** are *Worthy in His Eyes.*

What is Acquired Brain Injury?

Definition of Acquired Brain Injury

An acquired brain injury is defined as:

Damage to the brain, which occurs after birth and is not related to a congenital or a degenerative disease. These impairments may be temporary or permanent, and cause partial or functional disability or psychosocial maladjustment.

– World Health Organization (Geneva, 1996)

What Is Traumatic Brain Injury?

Traumatic brain injury is sudden physical damage to the brain. The damage may be caused by the head forcefully hitting an object such as the dashboard of a car (closed head injury) or by something passing through the skull and piercing the brain, as in a gunshot wound (penetrating head injury). The major causes of head trauma are motor vehicle accidents. Other causes include falls, sports injuries, violent crimes, and child abuse.

The physical, behavioral, or mental changes that may result from head trauma depend on the areas of the brain that are injured. Most injuries cause focal brain damage, damage confined to a small area of the brain. The focal damage is most often at the point where the head hits an object or where an object, such as a bullet, enters the brain.

In addition to focal damage, closed head injuries frequently cause diffuse brain injuries or damage to several other areas of the brain. The diffuse damage occurs when the impact of the injury causes the brain to move back and forth against the inside of the bony skull. The frontal and temporal lobes of the brain, the major speech and language areas, often receive the most damage in this way because they sit in pockets of the skull that allow more room for the brain to shift and sustain injury. Because these major speech and language areas often receive damage, communication difficulties frequently occur following closed head injuries. Other problems may include voice, swallowing, walking, balance, and coordination difficulties, as well as changes in the ability to smell and in memory and cognitive (or thinking) skills.

Specifically, acquired brain injuries are caused by:

TRAUMATIC FORCES TO THE HEAD WHICH CAUSE DAMAGE TO THE BRAIN

- Car crash
- Gunshot wounds to the head
- Objects falling on the head
- Falls
- Assaults

STROKE

- Embolism
- Thrombosis
- Aneurysm

BLEEDING IN THE BRAIN

- Intracranial surgery
- Hemorrhage
- Hematoma

LACK OF OXYGEN TO THE BRAIN

- Anoxia/hypoxia
- Near-drowning
- Cardiac arrest (heart stops beating)
- Drug overdose

INFECTIONS IN THE BRAIN

Toxic exposure

- Carbon monoxide poisoning
- Inhaling toxic chemicals
- Solvent sniffing
- Excessive and prolonged use of drugs and/or alcohol

Fluid build-up in the brain

Brain tumours

Acquired brain injuries can result in changes to how a person functions in the following areas:

Physical Changes
- Problems with walking, sitting, transfers, bathing, household tasks
- Slurred speech
- Chronic pain including headaches
- Fatigue and sleep difficulties

Cognitive Changes
- Takes more time to make sense of information
- Problems with planning, organizing or starting tasks
- Problems with vision
- Problems understanding conversations, coming up with the right word, talking in grammatically complete sentences
- Easily distracted
- Poor memory
- Difficulty with judgment and decision-making
- Preservation – "getting stuck" on a topic, idea or activity
- Confusion – may not know the date, year, time of day, where they are
- Impulsiveness – acting before you think
- Dis-inhibition – no "social filter" to tell you when you shouldn't do or say something

Emotional Changes
- Irritability "short fuse"
- Mood disorders like depression, anxiety, anger management problems
- Emotional liability – crying for no apparent reason
- Emotional or behavioural outbursts
- Normal emotional responses to the incredibly devastating impact of the brain injury
- Sadness, anger, frustration, loss of sense of self, anxiety about having another stroke or injury

SOCIAL CHANGES

- Awkwardness or inappropriate behaviour because of difficulty reading social cues
- Isolating yourself because you feel different, leading to being treated differently
- Trouble with social and work relationships because of awkwardness and poor coping skills
- Family breakdowns
- Loss of privacy, independence, future plans, income
- Change in roles (was a caregiver, now has to receive care from others)

Information obtained from:

POWELL RIVER BRAIN INJURY SOCIETY
Promoting prevention, recovery, education,
community awareness and life beyond brain injury.

EPILOGUE

GOD IS FAITHFUL

"However, as it is written: No eye has seen, no ear has heard,
no mind has conceived what God has prepared
for those who love him."
(1 Corinthians 2:9)

WRITING THIS BOOK HAS TAKEN SEVERAL YEARS, YET GOD NEVER removed the craving to share what I have within its pages. In fact, He intensified my desire to continue despite physical challenges of tremendous headaches and fatigue. Reviewing what I have written has been of tremendous encouragement to me. God continues to reveal many positive changes since November 7, 2001, strengthening my confidence, acceptance and contentment with who I am.

Reaching far beyond that personal revelation is the measureless hope available to every reader. To share God's incredible faithfulness with others is the very reason I fervently wanted to write this book. My heart yearns to encourage others who struggle in any area of life, whether you are experiencing difficulties that seem endless or hopeless, or whether you have a disability, visible or invisible.

As you read through this book, my prayer is that you will discover and embrace the indescribable love God the Father has for you, whatever your circumstances may be. I pray you will place your life in His divine care, permitting Him to turn your darkness into light, your fears into courage, and your hopelessness into hopefulness.

Above all, I urge you to trust and accept the Lord Jesus Christ as your personal Saviour. Doing so will bring lasting peace, deep and steadfast joy, and unwavering confidence in the worthiness of who you are. He will meet you *right* where you are. Just whisper His name. There is tremendous freedom and unshakeable security in the knowledge that you are a child of God. Your decision to accept Him as Lord guarantees life eternal.

Sharing my disability throughout these pages reveals my own personal struggles, experiences and victories, but each individual is unique and will carry different burdens. The point I want to stress is that none of us have to experience it or go through it alone; in fact, we mustn't do it alone. Self-focused determination can produce a temporary sense of success, and what we view as success through our own human efforts is nominal compared to what God can do in our lives when we place them in His total care.

We do not haphazardly wander through life without purpose. We didn't just happen to be. It is crucial to remember daily that our lives have been thought out from beginning to end, carefully shaped by God our Heavenly Father. Each life is so precious to Him that He sent His one and only Son to die on the cross so we could spend eternity with Him, an eternity free of tears, pain and sorrow. Armed with this truth, we can boldly lay claim to salvation and eternal life as children of God. Think about that for one moment. I am talking about Almighty God, the One Who has created the heavens, the earth and all contained therein! We have direct access to Him because of what Jesus did through shedding His blood on the cross! It is of eternal importance not to settle for *anything* less.

Accessing our loving God through His infallible Word and times of intimate prayer means we don't have to wonder about who is in control. We do not have to figure things out on our own! Yes, God calls us to be proactive with our life-choices, but trusting God completely dispels any darkness that may threaten to overpower us. That doesn't mean we will never experience difficulties, heartaches and pain, but it does guarantee we will not be overpowered by them as we rest securely in the Master's hand. Acts 17:24–25 says, *"The God who made the world and everything in it is the Lord of heaven and earth and does not live in temples built by hands. And he is not served by human hands, as if he needed anything, because he himself gives all men life and breath and everything else."* Verse 28 clarifies, *"For in him we live and move and have our being."*

Dependence on our own strength can magnify the reality of our human weaknesses. We will fall, we will fail, and we *will* end up in despair. But God wants us to experience victories, and He wants us to grow stronger in character. He expects us to use the gifts He has bestowed upon us individually; we are not a carbon copy of any other human being on this earth. More accurately, we are unique, priceless and valuable living treasures. You and I have been carefully and intricately moulded, created by Almighty God for a higher purpose which only we, individually, are qualified for.

Dependence on God does not display weakness. To depend on Him completely is to discover strength within that far surpasses our human efforts. Satan wants us to believe we can possess anything in the world we desire. He even tried to entice Christ with that same dangling carrot, but I caution you, he is the father of lies. Adam and Eve can certainly authenticate the harsh reality of Satan's lies. Paul warns us in 2 Corinthians 4:4, *"The god of this age has blinded the minds of unbelievers, so that they cannot see the light of the gospel of the glory of Christ, who is the image of God."* Satan, the god of this age, knows all too well the victories we can claim in Christ's name, rendering Satan useless.

I urge you to look beyond, far beyond what is humanly understandable. Discover what it means to fully trust Almighty God with your most precious asset, your life. "Surrender the chicken plate" so you can enter into a relationship with Christ that offers eternal hope. You may be required to become broken before the Lord, surrendering pride and heartaches at His feet. This is not a sign of weakness. It is the courageous first step of turning your life over to the One Who designed and created you, exactly as you are. No longer will you find yourself groping through the dark valley of hopelessness, for His Light will guide you to the exhilarating summit of possibilities and victories.

He offers hope. He offers abundant life. Your *circumstances* may not change, but your *heart* will. You will view difficulties and challenges from a much different perspective. You may even find the journey exciting! 1 Corinthians 2:9–10 says, *"However, as it is written: 'No eye has seen, no ear has heard, no mind has conceived what God has prepared for those who love him' but God has revealed it to us by his Spirit. The Spirit searches all things, even the deep things of God."*

I leave you with this beautiful passage of Scripture found in Romans 15:13,

> *"May the God of hope **fill** you with all joy and peace as you **trust in him**, so that you may **overflow** with hope by the power of the Holy Spirit"* (emphasis mine).

You *are* Worthy in His Eyes!